FREE
SPIRITED

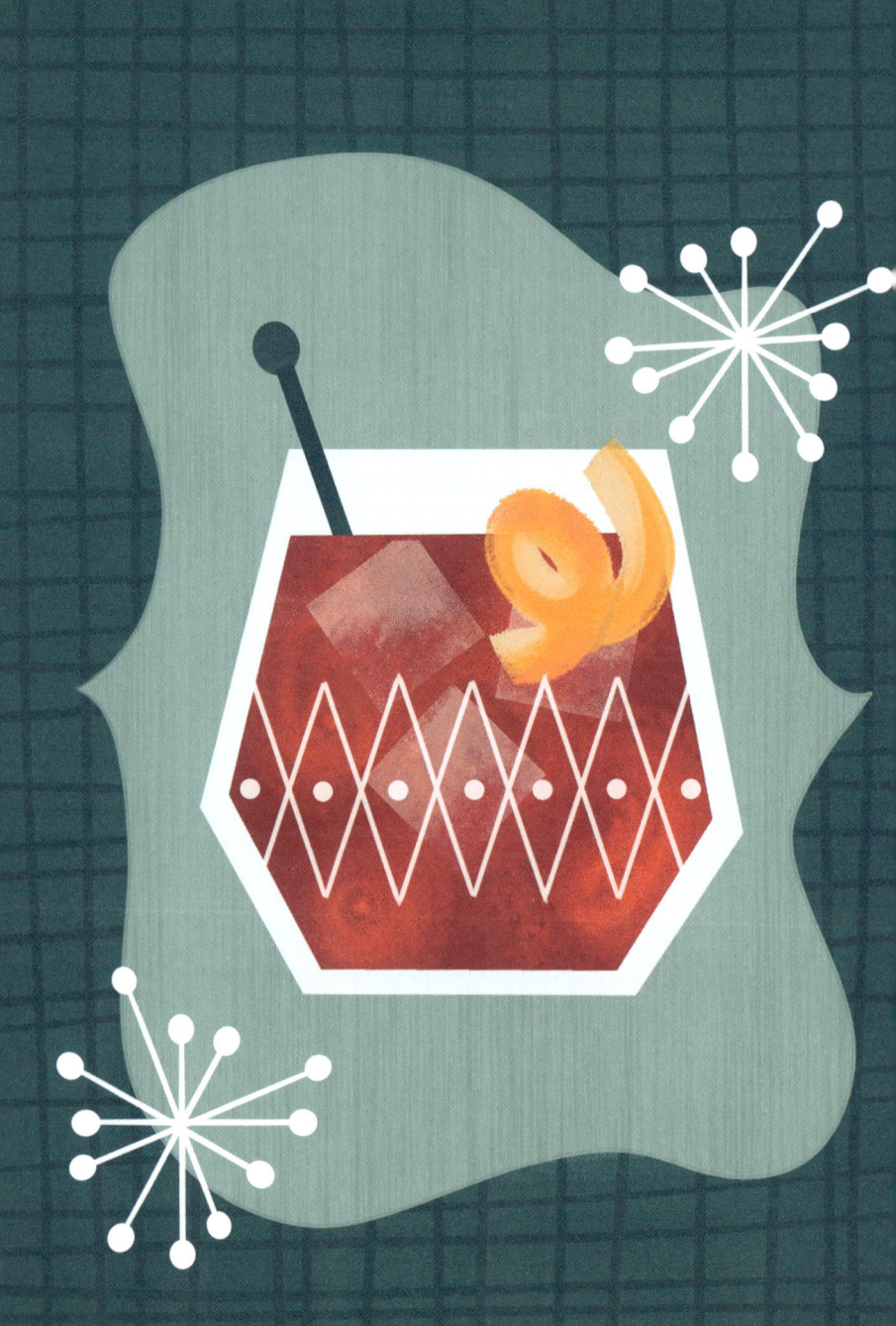

FREE
SPIRITED

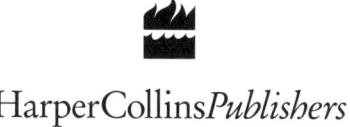

HarperCollins*Publishers*

HarperCollins*Publishers*

HarperCollins*Publishers*
1 London Bridge Street
London SE1 9GF

www.harpercollins.co.uk

HarperCollins*Publishers*
Macken House, 39/40 Mayor Street Upper,
Dublin 1, D01 C9W8, Ireland

First published by HarperCollins*Publishers* in 2024

1 3 5 7 9 10 8 6 4 2

Copyright © HarperCollins*Publishers* 2024

Written by Colleen Graham
Cover and interior images by Jaime Cromer
Cover design by Jacqui Caulton
Interior page design by Gareth Butterworth
Project editors: Sarah Varrow and Simon Holland

Colleen Graham asserts the moral right to be identified as the author of this work.

A catalogue record for this book is available from the British Library.

ISBN 978-0-00-866419-0

Printed and bound in Latvia

This book features recipes that include the optional use of raw eggs.
Consuming raw eggs may increase the risk of food-borne illness. Individuals
who are immunocompromised, pregnant, or elderly should use caution.
Ensure eggs are fresh and meet local food-standard requirements.

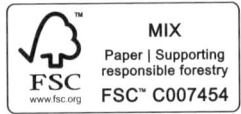

This book contains FSC™ certified paper and other controlled
sources to ensure responsible forest management.

For more information visit: www.harpercollins.co.uk/green

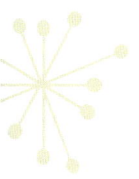

CONTENTS

FREE SPIRITED RECIPES

Free Spirited Classics

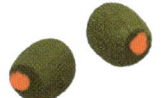

Free Spirited Innovations

WHAT MAKES A GREAT FREE-SPIRITED DRINK?

Cocktails versus mocktails – what is the difference? And what is a spirit-free drink? The answers require a bit of history. . .

The classic definition of a cocktail, established in the late 1800s, is a mixed drink that includes a liquor – or another alcoholic beverage, such as beer or wine – a bitter, a sweetener and water (typically in the form of ice). Bartenders have abided by this rule for over a century. Then, in the early 2000s, we drink writers grabbed onto the moniker 'mocktail'.

INTRODUCING MOCKTAILS

'Mocktail' is a play on the phrase 'mock cocktail', a mixed drink without alcohol. Crafty but simplistic! There have long been mocktail favourites such as the Shirley Temple, named after the iconic child actress, which became the go-to non-alcoholic drink in bars and restaurants. It took until the mid-2010s, however, for a mocktail movement to burst forth, leading to an entirely new market in the drinks industry.

As more people became conscious of how much they imbibed and the potential ill-effects of alcohol regarding their personal health and well-being, a growing interest formed in creating finer non-alcoholic beverages. You likely know of (amongst other catchy marketing slogans and hashtags) the 'Dry January' and 'Sober October' campaigns popping up on social media. People who give it a go being alcohol-free are often referred to as 'sober curious', which describes this approach and mindset. Those of us who specialized in crafting unique beverages started combining readily available ingredients (juices, nectars, sodas, etc.) to create fantastic mixed drinks, which would make anyone forget that there's no alcohol involved. And so began the mocktail revolution.

Today, they go by multiple names – non-alcoholic beverages, mocktails, zero-proof cocktails, no/lo cocktails and NA drinks – thanks to an innovative set of entrepreneurs who set out to recreate the taste of distilled spirits in a non-alcoholic form. What they achieved in so few years is astounding to veterans of this industry, and how we employ these new creations in drinks requires adaptation from everything we've practised for decades. A mock gin tastes like gin… but doesn't really taste like gin. It's an on-going enigma!

CREATING YOUR OWN DRINKS

Not every mocktail requires some replicated liquor. Several simply require a juice, sweetener, and sparkling beverage (and plenty of home-made mixers). Really, some of my best original mocktail recipes are incredibly simple! In *Free Spirited*, I hope you find the inspiration to continue your own drink pursuits – with no alcohol needed.

What I want to encourage most is to use the recipes in this book as a guide, a starting point for your own adaptations and experiments. No drink is ever 100 per cent perfect for 100 per cent of drinkers. Unlike baked goods that rely entirely on a specific formula in order to work out, mixed drinks should be adapted to your personal taste. I prefer a drier or tarter flavour, but if your taste goes more towards the sweet side, an extra dash of syrup will help. You're drinking it, I'm not.

In bartending, there are guidelines, tips, and tricks, but no concrete rules. Those men and women who have been slinging drinks behind the stick since the 1800s – putting in endless hours of work, honing their craft, and dealing with inebriated patrons of all sorts – left us a drinks-making legacy to honour and from which to learn. Whether you're shaking your first mocktail or are simply sober curious, we can all learn from their techniques, and then take it to the free-spirited world. Not every drink will be your thing, but the next one might. It's exciting.

So get in that kitchen, grab some sugar to make custom syrups, score that new zero-proof spirit that catches your eye at the shops and don't forget to stop by the produce section for fresh fruits and veggies! Have fun, enjoy the adventure, follow your taste, share it with those you love.

NAVIGATING
NO/LO SPIRITS

**Still relatively young, the market for zero-proof spirits is
evolving and growing. In my decades of experience in the
drink world, I have seen nothing like it.**

Gin, tequila and whisky have adhered to industry standards and taste
profiles for years – some laid out by territorial regulations. However,
this non-alcoholic spirits industry is a new game, and there are no
standards (yet) on how to approach zero-proof. The flavours and
production techniques vary greatly, and the only requirement is that
the company meets a standard of minimal (if any) alcohol within the
bottled product. NoLo or 'No/Low' has become the go-to term for
any beverages with no or minimal alcohol – especially as 'no alcohol' is
rarely absolute zero. In the UK and Europe, NoLo covers drinks under
1.2% alcohol. In the USA, 'no and low' must be used on labelling, as 0%
rarely means no alcohol is present, due to traces from fermentation
and distillation. So... industry standard and barspeak stick to 'NoLo'.

HOW DO YOU GET THE TASTE WITHOUT THE ALCOHOL?
It's extremely complicated, and a question I have asked many of the
non-alcoholic spirit producers. The answer is rarely the same. Some
distil the beverage in a similar way to alcoholic spirits, then remove
all (or most) of the alcohol. Others employ an infusion process that
requires no still or alcohol base. Zero-proof spirit producers generally
rely on botanicals to replicate the taste of liquors. Gin is an easy one
because it is a botanical-based, distilled spirit, so a variety of spices and
herbs are infused or distilled into the liquid. In the non-alcoholic market,
you'll see many of these labelled 'botanical spirits' (I use that name in
these recipes). While they are the most prevalent on the market, the
taste profile of these non-alcoholic gins varies greatly. Some have a
juniper-forward flavour similar to classically styled gin, while others
are softer and more floral, following what's called the 'New-world gin'
profile (such as that of Aviation and Hendrick's). Those with a softer

profile are an excellent substitute for vodka in cocktail recipes, adding a subtle floral twist. The non-alcoholic tequilas, rums and whiskies tend to use a robust spice of some kind to mimic the alcohol-enhanced flavour of those liquors. Some work well, but others require more sweetener in the recipe. Zero-proof spirits are not always great on their own. It's not like pouring a nice bourbon over ice or a two-finger pour of Scotch and sipping it straight – they need to be mixed. Non-alcoholic drinks makers encourage topping them with a soda or tonic to make a quick spritzer.

A FEW OF MY FAVOURITE BRANDS

Seedlip: This brand produces non-alcoholic botanical spirits with various flavour profiles, including spiced and floral options. This company was a front-runner in the zero-proof spirit market and offers nice options for gin and vodka substitutes.

Lyre's, Ritual, and Free Spirits: Probably boasting the most extensive portfolios, you could create an entire non-alcoholic bar with these zero-proof spirits, including gins, tequilas, rums, whiskies and aperitifs (including vermouth substitutes).

Optimist and Pentire: These brands offer more great substitutes for gin and vodka – with an array of flavour profiles.

Damrak Virgin: Produced by a great Dutch gin distiller, this is a really impressive zero-proof gin.

Three Spirits and Ghia: Both produce a series of botanical drinks that have a maltier mouth-feel. They could both act as substitutes for a dark spirit or liqueur.

Martini & Rossi: One of the best-known vermouth producers, it was really exciting when they released both non-alcoholic dry and sweet vermouths. Bring on those alcohol-free Martinis!

Fre: When searching for a non-alcoholic (technically 'alcohol-removed') wine, you'll find that this brand covers almost anything you need.

INGREDIENTS AND HOME-MADE MIXERS

With or without alcohol – what does every bar need? Incredible ingredients and an array of good mixers.

Beyond the zero-proof spirits, there are several essential mixers that you'll find invaluable in your free-spirited drink journey. Many of these you can buy, but several you can make from scratch at a fraction of the price. And, they're crazily easy to make once you know a few tricks!

SYRUPS

Many of my recipes call for a Simple Syrup, which, as the name implies, is very simple. It is the primary drink sweetener and really nothing more than sugar and water – seriously, that's it! This is the one ingredient I tell everyone not to buy, as it's a waste of money. Can you boil water and stir in a little sugar until it dissolves? Then you got this one! Plus, the flavour possibilities are only limited by the ingredients you have on hand – and your imagination.

I use flavoured syrups often – throughout the drink recipes – from Raspberry Syrup for a Raspberry Arnold Palmer (see page 74) to, my personal favourite, Lavender-honey Syrup for the Lavender Lemonade (see page 77).

Adding flavour to Simple Syrup is just as easy. All you need to do is add the desired flavouring ingredient to the sugar water, let it simmer, let it steep as the syrup cools, then strain out any solid ingredients. The longer you allow it to steep, the deeper the flavour evolves. It's a great way to add extra flavour to drinks and a substitute for flavoured liqueurs, including triple sec. Raspberries, herbs, citrus juice and zest, spices – they're all potential flavouring ingredients for your home-made syrups. You can also substitute a portion (usually half) of the water with any fruit juice. Have fun with this and think of interesting combinations that can elevate your drinks to new heights!

SIMPLE SYRUP

Makes about 350ml
400g white
  granulated sugar

To make a standard batch of Simple Syrup, bring 250ml water to a low boil in a small saucepan, then stir in the granulated sugar until dissolved. Reduce the heat, cover and simmer for about 5 minutes before removing it from the heat and allowing it to cool completely. When bottled (use a glass or plastic container with a tight seal) and refrigerated, Simple Syrup can last for up to 2 weeks.

VARIATIONS

• For a less sweet version than the 1:2 ratio, cut the sugar in half (200g).
• Rather than white sugar, use demerara sugar for a deeper, richer flavour. Brown sugar works, too.
• If you're looking to cut sugar and calories, there are options. Sugar alternatives can be tricky. After several experiments, I found that an allulose sweetener with monk fruit offers the best results; it has a universal taste that rivals traditional Simple Syrup. Avoid anything with erythritol and xylitol, as these crystallize once the syrup cools, and classic options like Sweet'N Low are simply too bitter for drinks.
• With any of these non-white, granulated sugar options, the ratio is generally the same – 200–400g sugar per 250ml water (adjusted to your ideal sweetness level, of course).

HONEY SYRUP

Makes about 350ml

840g honey

To make Honey Syrup, stir the honey with 250ml water until the honey dissolves; no boiling water is needed. Store in an airtight bottle or container in the fridge and use within 2 weeks.

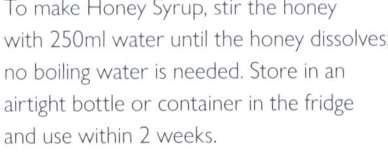

TIP

Honey that is runny and drips is easier to work with and dissolve. If your honey sets and becomes too thick, remove the lid and set the jar in hot water until it liquefies. You can also do this with small bursts in the microwave – at low power.

LAVENDER-HONEY SYRUP

Makes about 350ml

4 tbsp food-grade or
  culinary lavender buds
100g granulated sugar
280g honey

Bring 250ml water to the boil, add in the lavender buds and sugar and stir until the sugar has dissolved. Reduce the heat, stir in the honey and simmer for 10 minutes. Remove from the heat and allow to cool before straining out the lavender. It will keep for about 2 weeks, bottled, in the fridge.

ROSEMARY SYRUP

Makes about 350ml

400g white granulated sugar

3 tbsp fresh rosemary leaves or 1 tbsp dried rosemary

Bring 250ml water to a low boil, then stir in 400g white granulated sugar until dissolved. Add the rosemary, reduce the heat, cover and simmer for about 5 minutes before removing it from the heat and allowing it to cool completely. Strain, then bottle. Refrigerated and stored in an airtight bottle, Rosemary Syrup can last for up to 2 weeks.

ROSE SYRUP

Makes about 350ml

400g demerara sugar

115g culinary rosewater

Bring 250ml water to the boil, and stir in the demerara sugar until dissolved. Add the culinary rosewater, reduce the heat and simmer for about 10 minutes. Remove from the heat, cover and allow to cool completely before bottling. Store in an airtight bottle, refrigerate and use within 2 weeks.

SPICED BROWN SUGAR SYRUP

Makes about 350ml

200g soft brown sugar

2 cinnamon sticks

1 tbsp orange zest

1 tsp whole allspice

1 tsp cloves

1 tsp grated nutmeg

½ vanilla pod

Bring 250ml water to the boil and stir in the brown sugar until dissolved, then reduce the heat. Add the cinnamon, orange zest, allspice, cloves, grated nutmeg and vanilla pod. Simmer for 5 minutes, then remove from the heat, and allow to cool before straining and bottling. Store in an airtight bottle in the fridge for up to 2 weeks.

ORANGE SYRUP

Makes about 350ml

200g golden or white
  granulated sugar
grated zest of 2 navel
  oranges
2 tbsp grated, dried, bitter
  orange peel (optional)
1–2 tbsp freshly-squeezed
  orange juice (optional)

Bring 250ml water to the boil, and stir in
the sugar until dissolved. Add the orange
zest and dried peel, simmer on low for 5
minutes, then remove from the heat. Allow
to cool, then let it steep for at least 2 hours
(overnight is better if you have the time)
before straining out the citrus peels. If you
like, add a tablespoon or two of freshly-
squeezed orange juice. Once bottled, store
in the fridge for up to 2 weeks.

VANILLA-ORANGE SYRUP

Makes about 350ml

200g golden or white
  granulated sugar
1 vanilla pod, slit in half,
  or ½ tsp pure vanilla
  extract
Peel of 1 medium-sized
  orange

Bring 250ml water to the boil, and stir in
the sugar until dissolved. Add the vanilla
and orange peel, simmer on low for 5
minutes, then remove from the heat
and allow to cool. Store in the fridge for
up to 2 weeks – in a glass or plastic
container with a tight-fitting lid.

CINNAMON-ROSEMARY-MAPLE SYRUP

Makes about 350ml

115g pure maple syrup
1 rosemary sprig
1 cinnamon stick

Bring 250ml of water to a low boil, add the
pure maple syrup and stir until dissolved.
Add the rosemary sprig and cinnamon stick,
reduce the heat, and simmer for 5 minutes.
Remove from the heat, cover, and allow
to cool completely before removing the
rosemary and cinnamon and bottling. Store
in an airtight bottle or container in the
fridge for up to 2 weeks.

CINNAMON-LAPSANG SOUCHONG TEA SYRUP

Makes about 350ml
200g golden sugar
2 x 7.5-cm cinnamon sticks
lapsang souchong tea bag

Bring 250ml water to the boil, stir in the golden sugar until dissolved, then add the cinnamon sticks and a lapsang souchong tea bag. Simmer for 5 minutes. Remove from the heat, steep for 3–5 minutes, then remove the tea bag and let the cinnamon continue to infuse the syrup until cool. Once cool, remove the cinnamon sticks and bottle the syrup. Store in an airtight bottle or container for up to 2 weeks.

RASPBERRY SYRUP

Makes about 350ml
200g white granulated
  sugar
240g fresh or frozen
  raspberries

Bring 250ml water to a low boil, then stir in the white granulated sugar until dissolved. Once the sugar has dissolved, add the raspberries. Simmer for 5 minutes, and mash the raspberries as it simmers. Remove from the heat, and allow to cool completely before straining out the raspberries. Store in an airtight container or bottle, keep it refrigerated and use within 2 weeks.

SAGE SYRUP

Makes about 350ml
200g white, granulated
  or golden sugar
20g fresh sage leaves

Bring 1 cup water to the boil, stir in the sugar until dissolved and reduce to a simmer. Add the sage leaves, cover, and simmer for 5 minutes, then remove from the heat. Let the syrup cool completely, then bottle. Store in a bottle or airtight container in the fridge for up to 2 weeks.

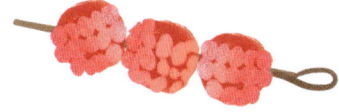

GRENADINE AND POMEGRANATE MOLASSES

Essential in classics such as the Shirley Temple (see page 78) and Roy Rogers (see page 109), grenadine is a very sweet, pomegranate-flavoured syrup that adds a brilliant red colour and fruity flavour to several drinks. Pomegranate molasses (or syrup) is not as sweet and typically includes a bit of citrus juice. The two can be used interchangeably, though the molasses is a touch more tart and definitely not as sweet as grenadine, so be sure to adjust your drinks to taste when using one for the other. To create a pomegranate syrup yourself, substitute all or half of the water in a Simple Syrup with pomegranate juice and a splash of lemon juice. Bottled pomegranate juice is good in this instance (possibly one of the few times I ever recommend it instead of using fresh ingredients), but it can be costly, so I tend to go with a 1:1 mix of juice and water. If you're in the mood for a winter kitchen project, when pomegranates are in season, go ahead and juice those little arils (it can get messy, so wear an apron), and make up the freshest pomegranate sweetener of the year!

DIY NON-ALCOHOLIC TRIPLE SEC

With its orange flavour, plus its sweet and semi-bitter taste, triple sec is one of the most commonly-used liqueurs for cocktails. Replicating it in non-alcoholic drinks is not difficult – just make an Orange Syrup (see page 16). The key to this essential, free-spirited substitute is bitter orange peel, which is available dried and best purchased from reputable spice companies.

CITRUS JUICES

Considering that citrus fruits are so readily available in markets, there is absolutely no reason to use anything other than freshly-squeezed juice in any drink. Lemon, lime and orange juices are often used as accent ingredients in cocktails, and you simply cannot get that same tart freshness from bottled juices. Take the time to squeeze juice – you can do it by the glass or squeeze a week's worth and store it in the fridge for up to 3 days. Your effort will pay off when you take that first sip of a well-crafted drink.

OTHER FRUIT JUICES

As with citrus fruits, all other fresh fruit juices are the preferred mixing options when working towards the best-tasting drinks. Admittedly, some fruits are easier to work with than others, so there may be times when you'll simply want to stop by the grocer's juice aisle to pick up a bottle. If you have an electric juicer, use it! Alternatively, toss fresh fruit flesh into a blender or food processor and give it a whirl (sometimes a splash of water will help the process). Then, you'll want to strain out the fruit pulp to create an easily mixable juice. For this, I typically line a fine-mesh sieve with a layer or two of muslin (it's not absolutely necessary, but creates a cleaner juice), then let the juice drip into a bowl, stirring the pulp periodically until it is as dry as possible.

HOME-MADE LEMONADE

A touch tart and a little sweet, home-made lemonade is a basic drink everyone can make, and it's the foundation for several recipes in this book. Make a full jug and keep it in the fridge, and you'll be ready to mix up a great mocktail any time it's needed. This basic formula works with other citrus fruits, too. Try it with limes, oranges, grapefruit or even pomelos to give your drinks a fun twist. For my home-made lemonade tips, fast-forward to the Watermelon Lemonade Spritzer recipe (see page 85).

FIZZY DRINKS

Using sparkling water, tonic or some other fizzy beverage – the sparkling effervescence of fizzy mixers can add a new life to your drinks. They come in all sorts of flavours (or just plain), and there are very few mixed drinks that cannot be enhanced with a splash or long pour of a fizzy liquid (go ahead and add one to almost any recipe in this book if you like – you'll receive no judgement here!).

Don't forget to look beyond the big, brand-name manufacturers. These drinks-making giants produce less-than-stellar beverages when compared with smaller, 'boutique' companies. They're often too sweet, artificially sweetened and flavoured with all sorts of unpronounceable ingredients you need a scientific degree to understand. Instead, seek out 'craft' fizzy drink producers. They tend to use natural ingredients, strive for flavour balance and make superior mixed drinks, giving you control over your beverage's final taste. While the craft fizzy drinks market is continually developing, two pioneers I can recommend are Q Drinks and Fever-Tree.

Sparkling water and soda water are essentially the same and very neutral in taste. Soda water tends to have a sweetener in the mix, while sparkling water is generally not as fizzy. You are free to use them as substitutes for each other, as you see fit.

Citrus fizzy drinks
Several drinks call for lemon-lime soda (think 7-Up and Sprite), but you can often get away with nearly any fizzy drink flavoured with citrus fruit as a substitute in recipes. Citrus fizzy drinks (such as a refreshing lemon-lime soda) can also be used in place of plain sparkling water or soda water – but remember that they are sweetened, so you'll want to cut the drink recipe's other sweetener a bit.

Cola
Oh, here's the kicker! The cola produced by Coca-Cola and Pepsi, which many of us grew up on, is not the real cola found in those old soda fountains poured by soda jerks as talented as any bartender. Artificial ingredients replaced the cola (or kola) nut flavouring in syrups years ago. Once you get a taste of the difference between those drinks and real cola, it's hard to drink the syrupy stuff again. Look out for bottles that use 'kola' or 'true cola' on the label or include kola nut in the ingredients list; these may not be common, but the companies that produce them are usually not shy about this fact. When using real cola, you may need to add a bit more sweetener to your mixed drinks.

Ginger ale and ginger beer
While both use ginger, there is a distinct difference. Ginger ale is sweeter and a great substitute for unflavoured or citrus fizzy drinks – it's pretty universal, so please start pouring! Ginger beer tends to be spicier, with a more pronounced ginger kick – this varies from one brand to the next, as some are definitely rather sweet.

Tonic
Tonic is probably my favourite type of soda water! I could drink tonic water straight all day and be very happy. Since it has a drier flavour profile, it is also very mixable and will play nicely off any beverage sweetener.

Home-made fizzy drinks

What is a 'soft' or fizzy drink? Carbonated water that is often both flavoured and sweetened. You can replicate many shop-bought options at home. Invest in a fizzy drinks machine that adds carbonation, use distilled or purified water, then add a flavoured Simple Syrup – and hey presto! You've created a fizzy beverage! With this simple formula to hand, you can replicate nearly any flavour available and have fun concocting your own.

The stand-out exceptions are Home-made Ginger Beer (see page 86) and tonic water. Commercially, the latter requires a complex array of aromatics, and extracts quinine (responsible for the dry, bitter taste) from cinchona bark. Since there is a toxicity issue with that particular ingredient, and as it requires scientific precision, I suggest only following recipes that are quinine-free. We won't share any in this book, but it is a fun way to create your own customized tonic water.

Bitters

Cocktail bitters are concentrated, flavoured mixers that are used to add a subtle but necessary punch of flavour to drinks. Bitters have an alcohol base, but only a dash or two is required – so, as each drink has only a trace of alcohol, the result remains a genuine mocktail. Aromatic and orange bitters are the most common flavours, but you can have fun with others, such as cherry, chocolate, grapefruit, rhubarb – or even walnut. You'll find bitters in the Stay Sober Old Fashioned (see page 44) and No-groni (see page 56) – and I encourage you to use them for other drinks, particularly any 'tinis' and short drinks you care to design.

Now is the time to choose. Take a tour of the recipes – the Classics and the Innovations – and savour every step on your free-spirited journey.

CLASSICS

ZERO-PROOF MARGARITA

The margarita is among the quintessential drinks of the cocktail world, and it's surprisingly fabulous without tequila. All you really need is a trio of citrus juices (lime, of course, with a bit of orange and lemon) and a little sweetener. This Zero-proof Margarita is just that little bit more refreshing thanks to a fizzy touch – delivered by either sparkling water or soda water. The result is a lime-forward, thirst-quenching mocktail that rivals any tequila drink. This version is best shaken and served on the rocks, so be sure to have plenty of ice cubes ready in the freezer.

Serves 1

2 lime wedges, for the
  rim and to garnish
sea salt flakes or margarita
  salt for the rim
ice cubes
60ml freshly-squeezed
  lime juice
30ml freshly-squeezed
  lemon juice
30ml freshly-squeezed
  orange juice
15ml agave nectar
60–120ml sparkling water
  or soda water, to taste

Wipe the rim of a rocks or highball glass with one of the lime wedges, then roll or dip the rim in a small dish filled with the salt of your choice. Into a cocktail shaker filled with the ice cubes, add the lime, lemon and orange juices, and the agave nectar. Shake well, then strain into the rimmed glass filled with fresh ice cubes. Top with sparkling or soda water and garnish with the second lime wedge.

VARIATION

Want to make a non-alcoholic margarita with a zero-proof tequila? Use 45ml zero-proof tequila, 30ml Orange Syrup (see page 16), and 20ml lime juice. Shake it and strain it over crushed ice.

PERFECT MOJITO

Ah, the mojito. . . One of summer's favourite drinks! And if your garden includes mint, then you're ready to make a round of mojitos any time the mood suits you. Nothing more than a sparkling drink with rum, mint and lime, the mojito is really easy to make without alcohol – simply skip the rum! Of course, you can add a zero-proof rum if you like, but this drink is just as refreshing without it. I have found that using Honey Syrup makes a significant difference, adding a dark, sweet taste, which makes up wonderfully for the lack of rum. Simple Syrup will also do, and you can certainly play around with home-made flavoured syrups (any citrus works really well). Also, the fizzy element is up to your taste; sparkling water (plain or flavoured), citrus fizzy drinks and even tonic can make for an interesting mojito. Toss a few berries into the muddle, or some other fruit that's in season. There really are no rules with the mojito!

Serves 1

1 lime, cut into 4 wedges
30ml Honey Syrup
  (see page 14) or Simple
  Syrup (see page 13)
10 fresh mint leaves, torn
ice cubes
120–180ml soda water,
  sparkling or tonic water
1 fresh mint sprig,
  to garnish

Place three lime wedges, the syrup and the torn mint leaves into a highball glass. Muddle well to release the citrus juice and mint essence. Fill the glass with the ice, top with soda water, then stir. Garnish with the fourth lime wedge and the sprig of mint.

VARIATIONS

If you'd like to try adding a shot of non-alcoholic rum, you'll likely want to add a bit more syrup. Approximately 30ml rum with an extra 7ml syrup is about perfect.

VIRGIN BLOODY MARY

In the spirit of keeping everything ultra-fresh, the Virgin Bloody Mary is best made from scratch. All you need are a few store-cupboard staples and tomato juice, along with some fun garnishes. The blend of lemon, Worcestershire sauce, celery salt, black pepper and hot sauce is the perfect seasoning combination for tomato juice. It works perfectly well with a bottled tomato juice (avoid the canned stuff – it's just not great), so all you need to do is pour and stir. However, I do also encourage you to try this with fresh tomato juice at least once. Processing tomatoes into juice is just like making tomato sauce, but you don't simmer it down. Simply blanch and peel the tomatoes, run them through a food mill or blend them in a blender, then strain and refrigerate. You can even freeze the juice for later, and the fresher taste is so worth it.

Serves 1

120–150ml fresh or
    bottled tomato juice
    (see headnote)
15ml freshly-squeezed
    lemon juice
dash Worcestershire sauce
pinch celery salt
pinch freshly ground
    black pepper
2 dashes hot sauce
    (try Tabasco or Cholula),
    or to taste
ice cubes
1 celery stick,
    pickle spear, and lemon
    wedge, to garnish

Pour the tomato juice into a tall glass, and add the lemon juice, Worcestershire sauce, celery salt, pepper and hot sauce. Fill the glass with the ice and stir really well (don't skimp on this step; the ice dilution softens the taste of the tomato). Taste and add a few more dashes of hot sauce, if you like, then add the garnishes.

VARIATION

Try this drink with fresh cherry tomatoes. The tomato juice yield is smaller, so you'll likely want to use a double old-fashioned glass and cut the seasonings in half. Muddle about six cherry tomatoes in the glass to extract all of their juice, add the seasoning, fill with ice, then stir well.

BELLINI SPARKLER

When it's time for a celebration, the sparkling wonder that is the Bellini is an ideal choice. Peachy, effervescent and made from just two ingredients. . . How could you pass this one up? Typically made with Prosecco, the Bellini Sparkler opts for sparkling cider instead. The real secret is to ensure the ingredients and glasses are well chilled. Its peach component is typically peach nectar, of which there are several brands available. You can also use peach juice or a purée (both available commercially, though also easy to make at home). The purée is a bit thicker, but makes a lovely drink nonetheless. And, if you have the juice, you can make peach nectar by adding a sweetener and lemon or lime juice to taste. If you opt for the peach slice garnish, be sure to squeeze some lemon juice over it as soon as it is cut. This is one of those fruits that oxidizes and turns brown rather quickly. I like a squeeze of lemon juice in the Bellini, so a lemon wedge is also a great finishing touch.

Serves 1

60ml peach nectar, juice
    or purée, chilled
    (see headnote)
120–150 non-alcoholic
    sparkling cider, chilled
squeeze of juice from
    lemon wedge (optional)
1 peach slice, to garnish

Pour the cold nectar and cider into a chilled Champagne flute. Add the squeeze of lemon and garnish with the peach slice.

VARIATIONS

Try the Bellini Sparkler with ginger ale or another fizzy drink in place of the cider. This drink really needs a lot of carbonation (that's what mixes the ingredients). Some sparkling waters might not have enough fizz to pull that off, so you might need to give the drink a quick stir. Also, have fun with cucumber, citrus, lavender or vanilla fizzy drinks – each can be really interesting when set against the peach.

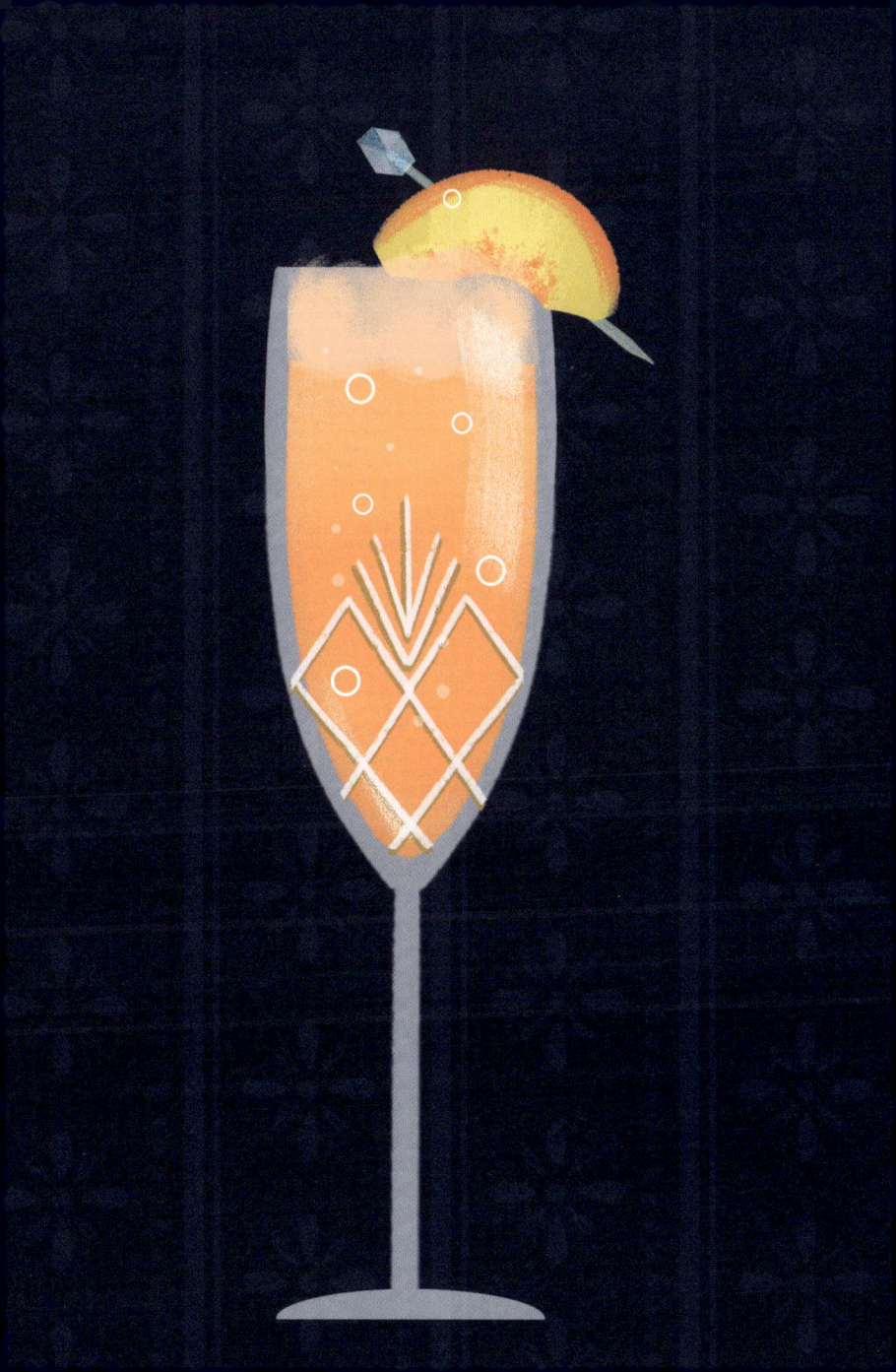

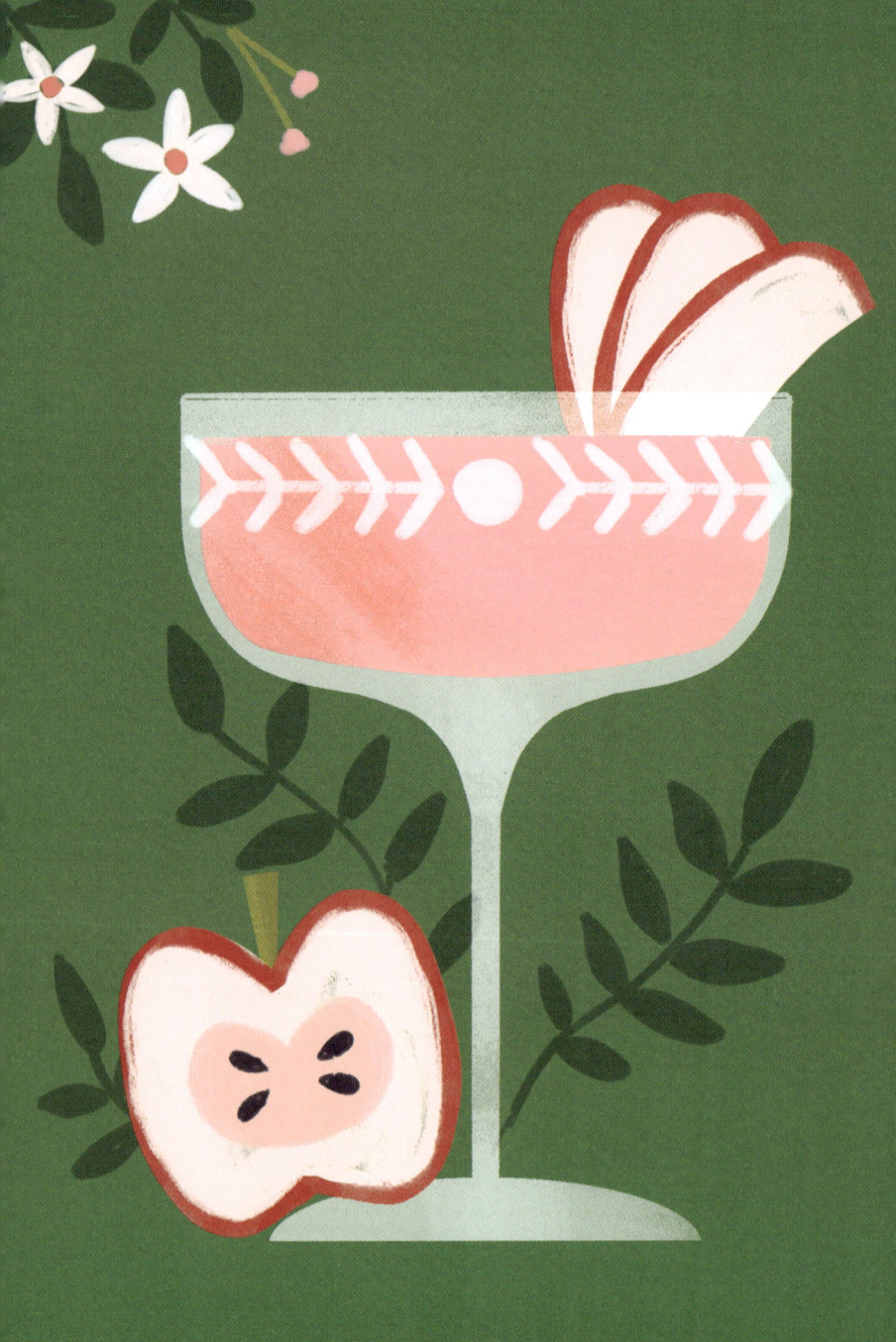

DESIGNATED APPLETINI

This mock Apple Martini relies on fresh apple juice, as, honestly, the bottled stuff is not all that great – though it is an option in a pinch. If you can make fresh apple juice (see Tip for guidance), you will have one divine Appletini. To make it extra special, rim the glass. In the autumn, I like a cinnamon-sugar rim (1 part ground cinnamon and 2 parts sugar), but white sugar alone works great year-round. Also, remember to squeeze lemon juice over the apple slices so they stay beautiful.

Serves 1

1 lemon wedge, for
  the rim
cinnamon sugar or white
  sugar, for the rim
120ml fresh or bottled
  apple juice (see Tip)
15ml Simple Syrup
  (see page 13)
½ tbsp freshly-squeezed
  lemon juice
ice cubes
apple slices, to garnish

Wipe the rim of a cocktail glass with the lemon wedge, then roll or dip the rim in a small dish filled with the sugar of your choice. In a cocktail shaker, add the apple juice, syrup and lemon juice. Fill with the ice and shake well. Strain into the prepared glass and garnish with the apple slices.

TIP

Working in batches, wash and quarter a tub of apples, then place them in a pot with just enough water to cover. Boil for 10 minutes or so until soft, then run them through a food mill to remove the skins. Finally, run the pulpy mix through a fine-mesh sieve. The juice will collect in the bowl, while the sieve holds fresh apple purée. Both elements can be frozen in plastic, freezer-safe bags for up to a year, and thawed as required.

SWEET SUNRISE

The Sweet Sunrise is really nothing more than a Tequila Sunrise, hold the tequila. It's an incredibly simple orange juice drink that's sweetened with grenadine. While a relatively basic beverage, it is a fantastic option for breakfast or brunch, and the sweet pomegranate-flavoured syrup offsets some of the orange juice's acidity, making it an easy drinker. For years, I made this drink with just the two ingredients – still a great option. After the introduction of zero-proof tequilas, I gave it another try. The non-alcoholic spirit adds a bit more depth to the drink, with an herbal tone that mimics the essence of real tequila. Add the spirit if you like, or don't. Either way, don't stir this one after adding the syrup or you'll lose the sunrise effect. The point of any sunrise is to enjoy its visual appeal, allowing the sweetness to rise, slowly, as you sip.

Serves 1

ice cubes
45ml non-alcoholic tequila
  (optional)
120–180ml orange juice,
  preferably freshly
  squeezed
15–30ml grenadine,
  to taste
1 orange slice, to garnish

Add the ice to a highball glass, pour in the tequila and orange juice and stir well. Slowly drizzle the grenadine over the drink; it will sink. Avoid stirring any further. Garnish with the orange slice and enjoy.

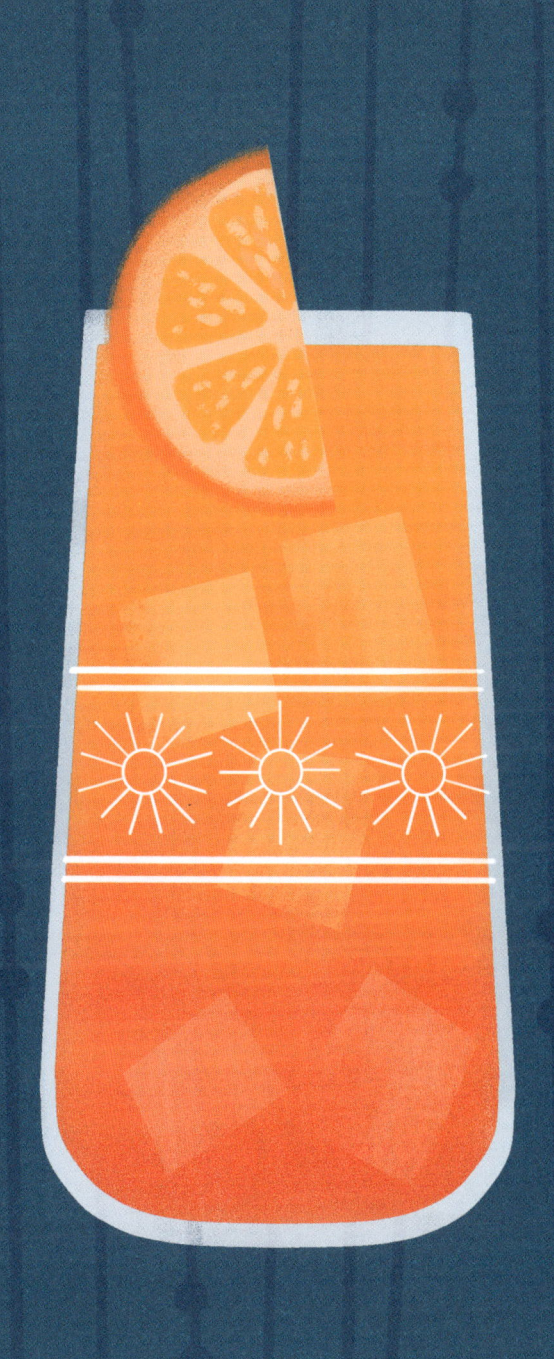

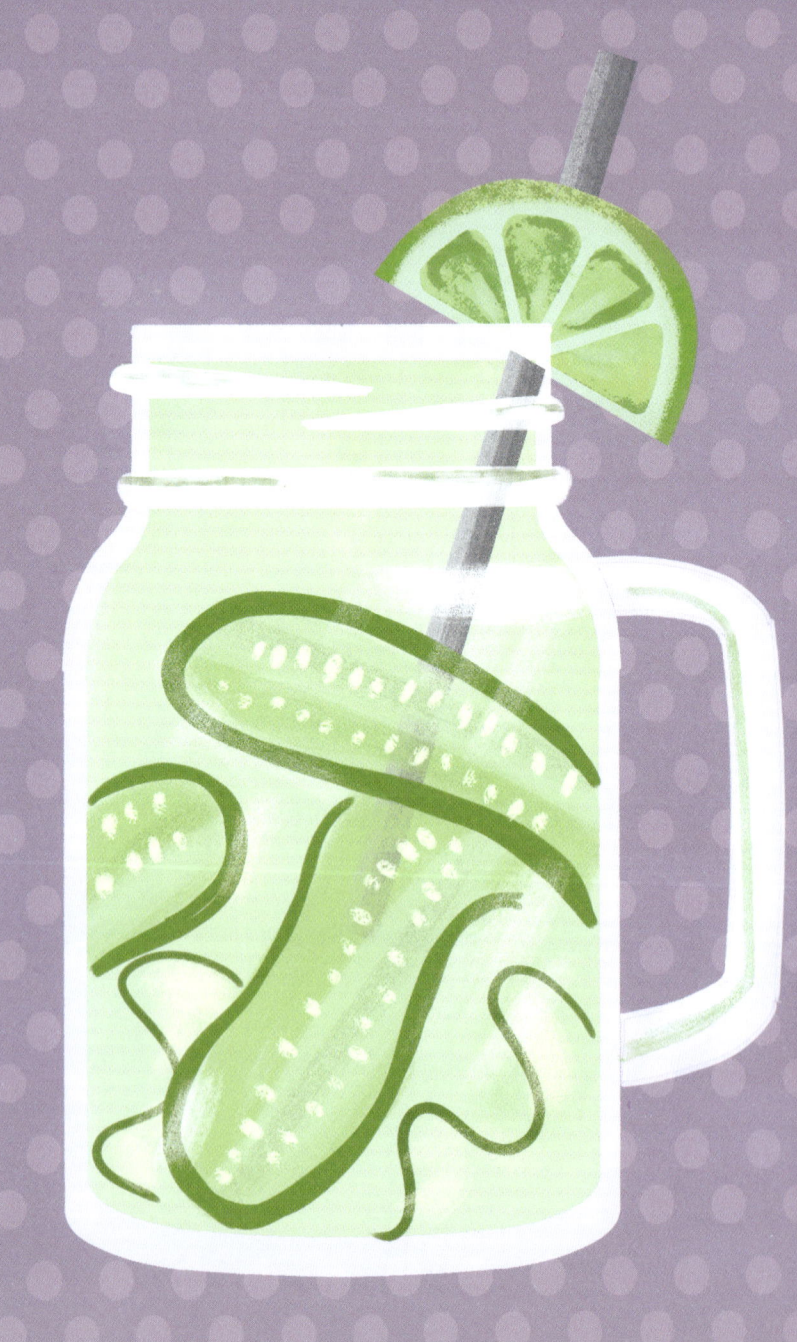

CUCUMBER COLLINS

While it's certainly not as common as citrus fruits or berries, the cucumber is an important ingredient to have in your cocktail/mocktail arsenal. If you have not enjoyed this experience, once you get a taste for its clean, ultra-refreshing flavour, you will certainly find more than one way to utilize it. The Cucumber Collins is the ideal place to begin. The original version uses gin, but in the free spirited world, a botanical non-alcoholic spirit will do just fine. Since that market is so diverse, this mocktail is a great way to explore your options because it is so clean and refreshing. I've found that the non-alcoholic spirits with softer botanical flavors – such as lavender – are the most pleasant, as they pair nicely with the cucumber and lime (see Navigating No/Lo Spirits, pages 10–11). Seeds in drinks are not very desirable, so opt for a seedless cucumber or remove any large seeds you find. Before slicing, run a vegetable peeler along the outside of the cucumber to create a few long, thin slices to weave within the ice. It's a simple trick with a dramatic effect, and will infuse more flavour into the mocktail.

Serves 1

2 slices cucumber
2 lime wedges or
  half wheels
30ml Simple Syrup
  (see page 13)
45ml zero-proof gin or
  non-alcoholic botanical
  spirit
ice cubes
90–120ml sparkling water
  or soda water, to taste
2–3 cucumber ribbons and
  1 lime slice, to garnish

In a cocktail shaker, muddle the cucumber and lime wedges (or half wheels) with the Simple Syrup. Add the non-alcoholic botanical spirit, fill the shaker with some ice cubes and shake well. Weave cucumber ribbons around the inside edge of a highball glass, then add some ice cubes. Strain the shaken mix into the glass, then top with the sparkling water or soda water, and garnish with the lime slice.

VIRGIN PIÑA COLADA

This recipe is a simple variation on a classic frozen Piña Colada. If you have no-proof rum on hand, add it! However, it's just as delicious without the rum (it will create a slightly shorter drink; add a couple of extra ice cubes or a splash of pineapple juice, if needed, to create a balanced drink). Since rum alternatives are not as sweet as the real liquor, a splash of Simple Syrup may be needed. Cream of coconut is the go-to ingredient for any kind of colada. It's sweetened and just the right consistency for blending into drinks; look for it in the mixers section at off-licences. Coconut cream is different. You get the same flavour without the sweetener (although some are sweetened, so read the label), but the cream is much thicker. If you have unsweetened coconut cream, add 1 to 2 tablespoons of Simple Syrup or honey. As with all non-alcoholic adaptations of popular cocktails, taste the mix after the first blending – and adjust and re-blend as desired.

Serves 1

60ml non-alcoholic
  rum (optional)
7.5–15ml Simple Syrup
  (optional, see page 13)
30ml pineapple juice
30ml cream of coconut
  or coconut cream
  (see headnote)
7.5–15ml freshly-squeezed
  lime juice, to taste
200g ice cubes
1 pineapple wedge and
  maraschino cherry,
  to garnish

Add the ingredients to a blender and blend until smooth. Pour into a tall, chilled glass and garnish with the pineapple wedge and cocktail cherry.

VARIATIONS

Toss 125g or so of frozen pineapple cubes into a blender, and halve the pineapple juice and ice quantities. Coconut milk will work here as well; preferably full-fat. The drink won't be as luscious as it is with cream of coconut, and you'll want to add a sweetener – as you would with coconut cream if it's unsweetened. A little extra ice or frozen pineapple will thicken the mix.

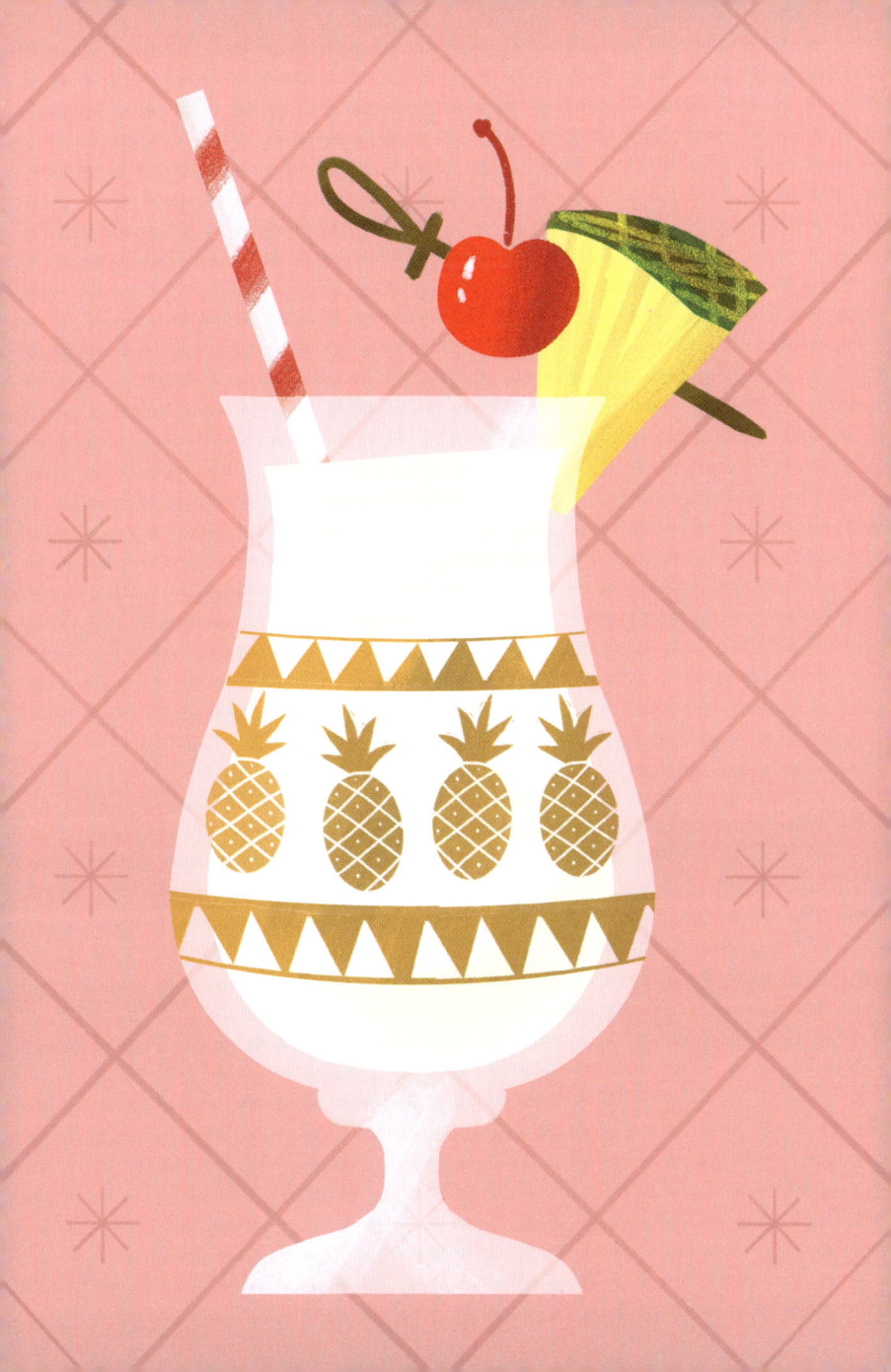

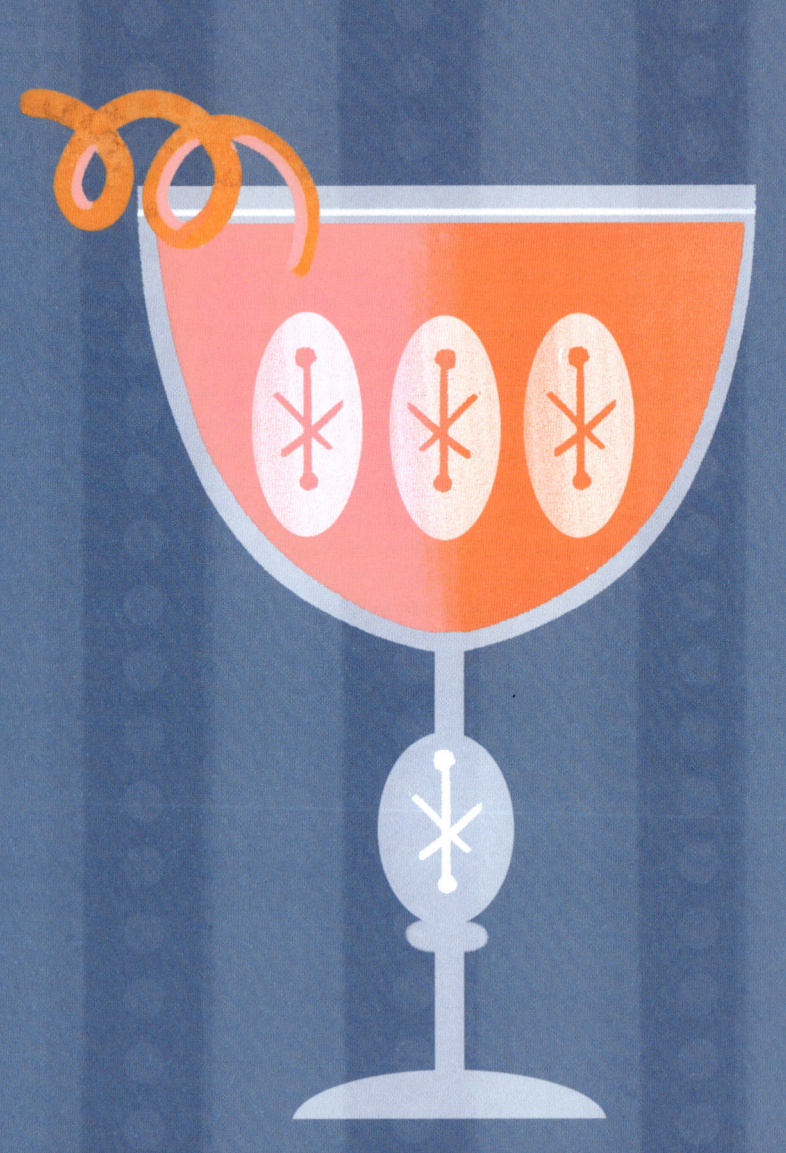

COS-NO-POLITAN

Call it a Cosmopolitan or a Cosmo; by either name, it's one of the most popular fruit Martinis in the world. It's really a simple mix – vodka, triple sec and lime and cranberry juices – and it's an easy sipper. While the Cosmo's origins go back as far as the early twentieth century, its popularity soared when it became the drink of choice for the ladies of *Sex and the City*. How do you transform this pretty, blush-pink Vodka Martini into a non-alcoholic delight? Turn to the lightly-flavoured, non-alcoholic botanical spirits designed to replicate gin and choose one with a delicate botanical profile for best results (if you have one with a bolder taste, add more cranberry juice). You'll definitely want to make a triple sec substitute for this drink, such as the Orange Syrup, though an orange-flavoured Simple Syrup is a good alternative. Fresh lime juice is utterly essential – don't skimp here! In the vodka-laced version, many of us prefer less cranberry to create a drier drink (a pale, transparent pink colour rather than a rosy red), but the Cos-no-politan is actually a bit better with more cranberry. However, it's all going to depend on the zero-proof spirit you have on hand. This is definitely a drink that should be adapted with each bottle in your explorations.

Serves 1

45ml zero-proof
  gin or non-alcoholic
  botanical spirit
30ml non-alcoholic triple
  sec or Orange Syrup
  (see page 16)
15ml freshly-squeezed
  lime juice
15–30ml cranberry juice
ice cubes
1 orange twist, to garnish

Pour the ingredients into a cocktail shaker filled with the ice – and shake vigorously. Strain into a chilled cocktail glass and garnish with the orange twist.

VARIATION

Fruit juice blends that include cranberry are fun ways to switch up the recipe. Cranberry-pomegranate is a particular favourite, but feel free to experiment with others.

LEMON DROP MARTINI MOCKTAIL

Simultaneously sweet and tart, the Lemon Drop is a taste sensation, making it an excellent dessert cocktail. Like the Cosmopolitan, it's an extremely popular Vodka Martini that requires similar adaptations when bringing it into the spirit-free realm. The Lemon Drop Martini Mocktail also needs a softly-flavoured, non-alcoholic botanical spirit to replace the vodka. Seek out those with florals, such as lavender and rose, along with a dominant citrus profile. Try to avoid any that have juniper or too many spices that try to replicate gin, as they'll overpower the delicate balance of sweet lemon in this drink. The essentials in any Lemon Drop are fresh lemon juice and Simple Syrup. As a final touch, the sugared rim gives this mocktail its spectacular, candy-like identity.

Serves 1

1 lemon wedge
granulated sugar, for
   the rim
60ml softly-flavoured,
   zero-proof gin or non-
   alcoholic botanical spirit
30ml freshly-squeezed
   lemon juice
15–20ml Simple Syrup
   (see page 13), to taste
ice cubes
1 lemon slice, to garnish

Wipe the rim of a cocktail glass with the lemon wedge. Roll or dip the rim in a small dish filled with the sugar. Pour the liquids into a shaker filled with ice, shake vigorously, then strain into the prepared glass. Garnish.

VARIATIONS

Try creating a strongly-flavoured, lemon-infused Simple Syrup that's similar to the ultra-sweet, citrus taste of limoncello. Use 250ml water and 200g sugar with the zest of an entire lemon and about 60ml fresh lemon juice. It should be too sweet and tart to drink straight, but that's okay because you're mixing with it.

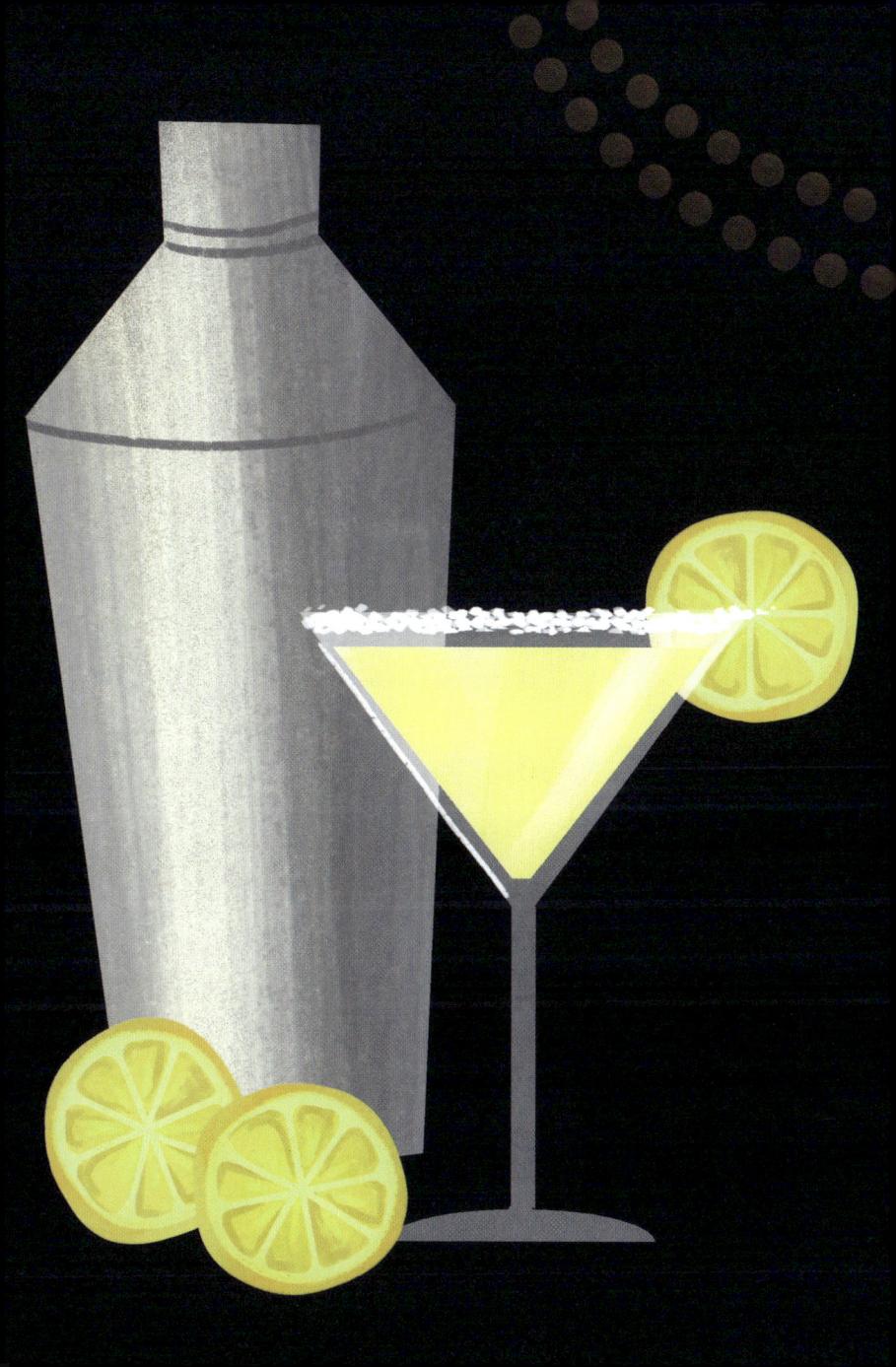

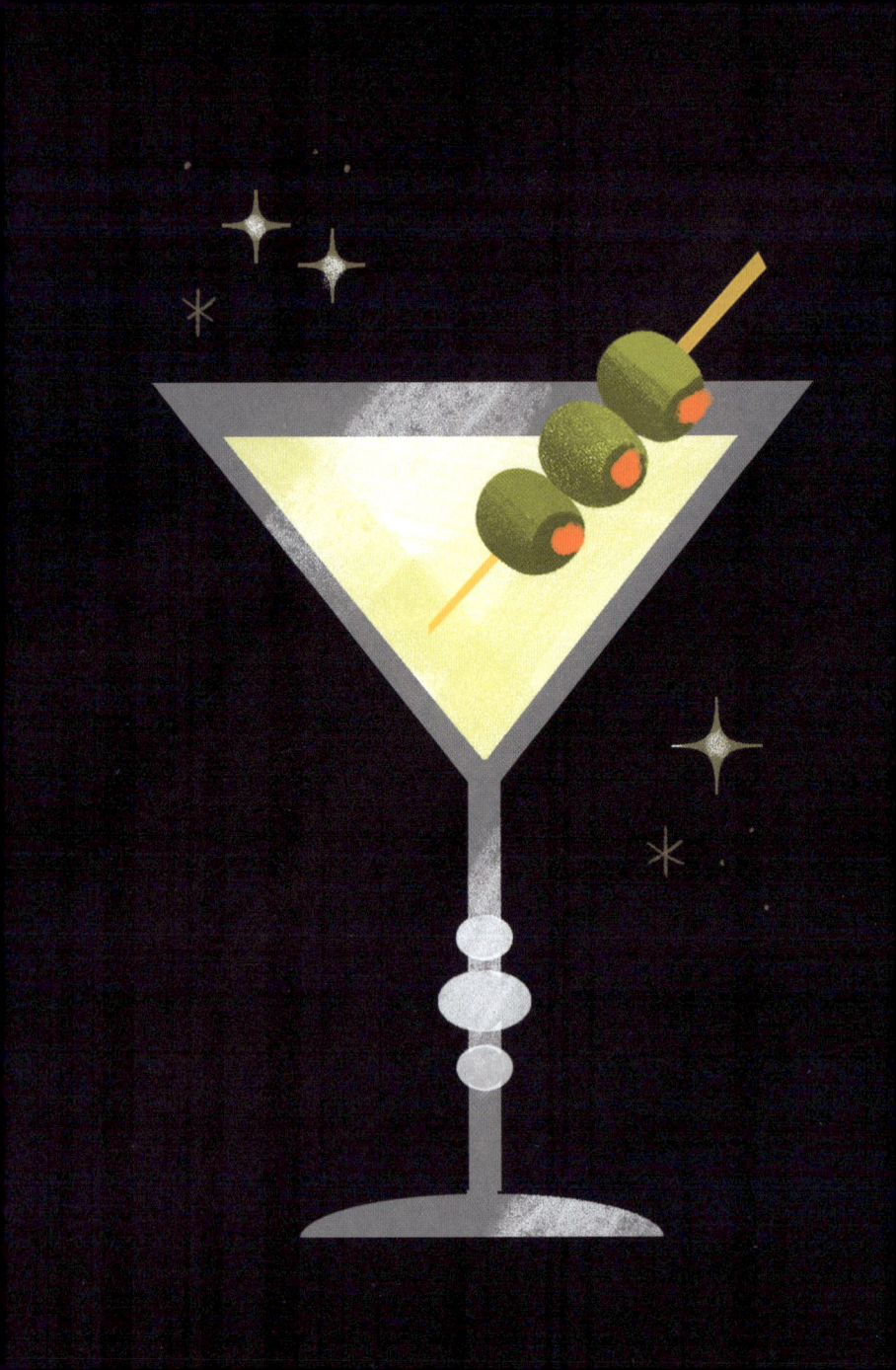

MOCK MARTINI

To make a Mock Martini, you want to consider the original cocktail's two elements separately. Explore various combinations and change the ratio from the suggested 2:1 to create a well-balanced drink that suits your taste. Zero-proof gin and other non-alcoholic botanical spirits are the most plentiful variety in the non-alcoholic spirits industry. For this drink, seek out those with a juniper-forward flavour; you'll even find some that indicate they're a 'London dry' alternative, and that's the best bet for a classic gin taste. Lightly-flavoured spirits are a better option if you like Vodka Martinis. Vermouth has also been replicated as 'aperitifs', and the array of flavour profiles available can be even more complicated to navigate. Some brands specifically mention vermouth in the name, while others stick to 'aperitif'. Keep in mind that there are dry and sweet vermouths; for a classic dry Martini, look for bottles that mention a dry profile. The other element to any Martini is the garnish. Go with a large olive (or skewer 3 smaller olives) or use this as an excuse to practise creating the perfect lemon twist. Either will infuse the drink with more flavour, so try to avoid skipping this simple step.

Serves 1

60ml zero-proof gin or non-alcoholic botanical spirit
30ml non-alcoholic dry aperitif, or to taste
ice cubes
2–3 dashes orange or aromatic bitters (optional)
1 or 3 olives or lemon twist, to garnish

Pour the two spirits into a cocktail shaker filled with ice. Stir for at least 30 seconds to add dilution and soften the flavour. Strain into a chilled cocktail glass, add bitters if you like, and garnish with the olives or lemon twist.

VARIATION

To make a Mock Dirty Martini, add a splash of olive juice. This works best with classic 'London dry' style zero-proof gins and 'dry' aperitifs. An olive garnish is most definitely required!

STAY SOBER OLD FASHIONED

One aspect I enjoy about non-alcoholic iterations of whisky, is that many tend to have the spicy aspect of rye whisky. It's the original whisky style used in an Old Fashioned. In this drink, which can be traced back to the 1850s, there is a hint of citrus and sweetener with the punch of bitters to soften the whiskey 'kick'. That's really the point of the Old Fashioned – you want a stiff whisky drink that's a little tamer. It's an incredibly easy drink, and infinitely adaptable to the whisky at hand. In the Stay Sober Old Fashioned, you can get that same taste sensation of spice, bitterness, citrus and sweetness. I add a little more sugar and recommend adapting this recipe to the zero-proof whisky that you're pouring at the moment. While the classic Old Fashioned doesn't include orange in the muddle (that's more of a modern twist), it mellows the mock-whisky's flavours. This is a drink you'll want to serve over the largest chunk of ice you can fit in your glass. As it melts, the diluting effect of the ice softens the mocktail as you enjoy it – sip by sip.

Serves 1

½ tbsp Simple Syrup
   (see page 13)
3 dashes aromatic or
   orange bitters
1 orange slice
ice cubes
60ml zero-proof whisky
1 orange twist and fresh
   or maraschino cherry,
   to garnish

Add the Simple Syrup, bitters and orange slice to an old-fashioned glass. Muddle well to incorporate the ingredients and release juice from the orange. Fill the glass with the ice, add the non-alcoholic whisky and garnish with the orange twist and cherry.

VARIATIONS

The classic Old Fashioned uses a sugar cube rather than a syrup. Go that route if you like, or use ½ to ¾ teaspoon white or raw granulated sugar in the muddle.

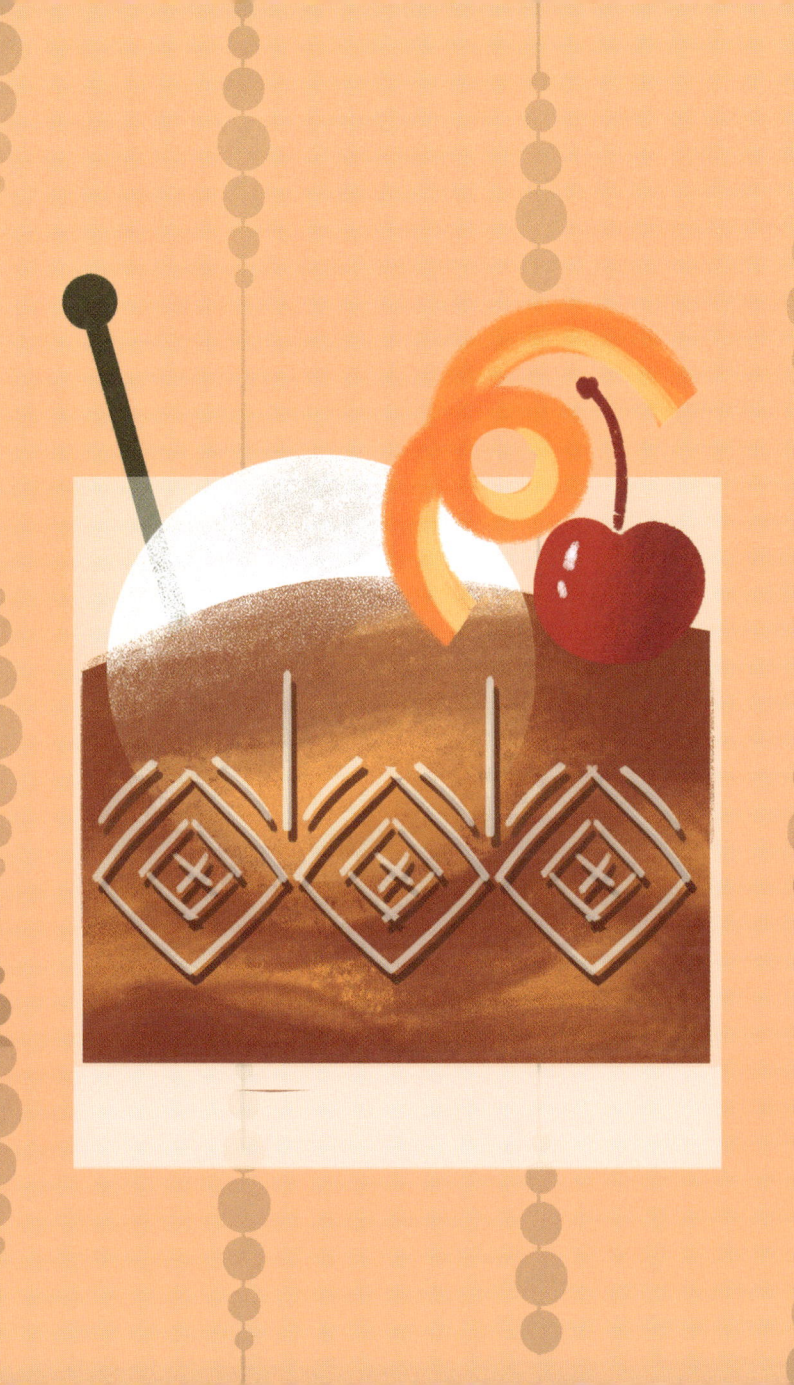

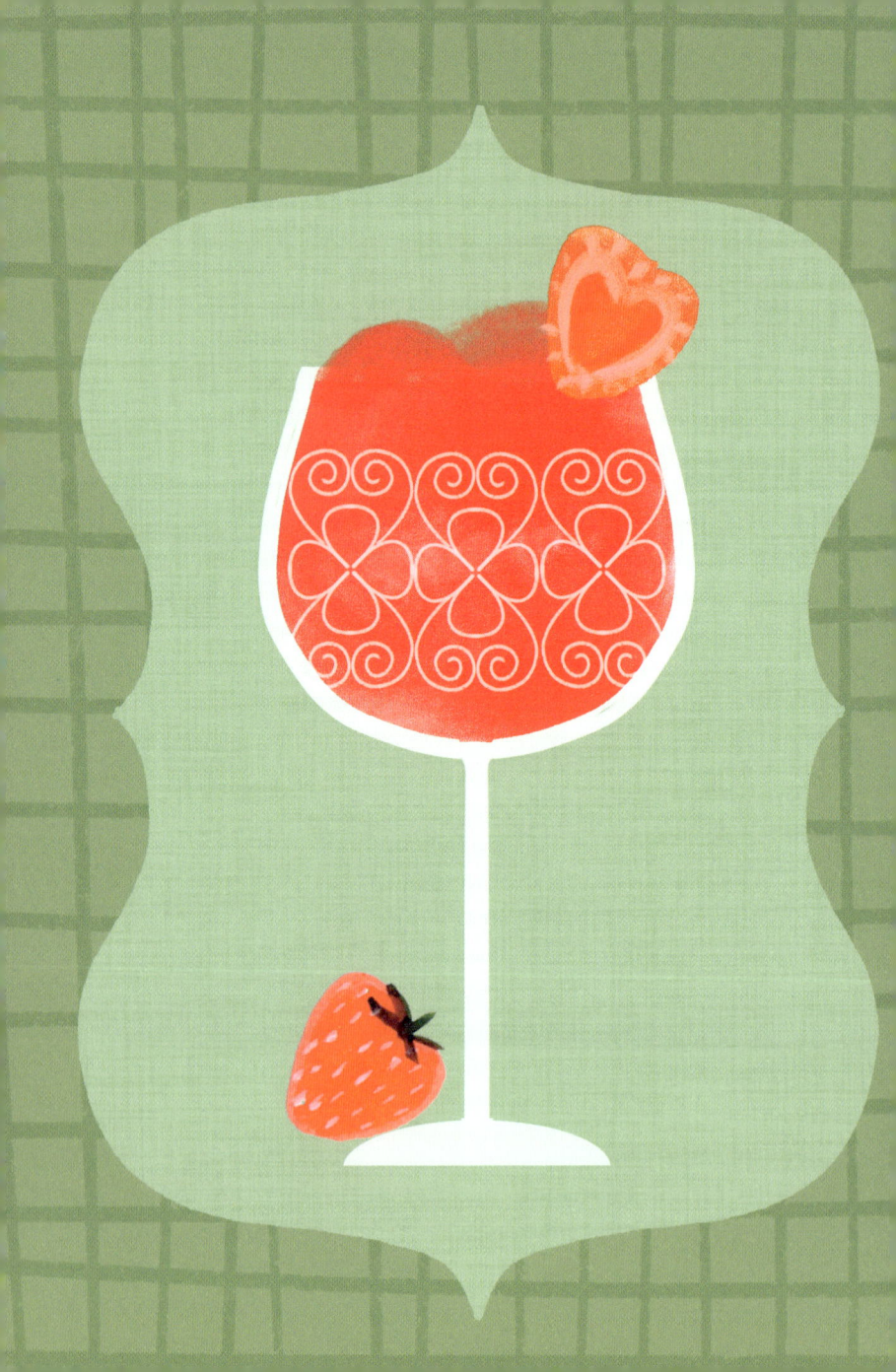

SKIP THE ROSÉ FROSÉ

The Frosé is the ultimate wine-based slushie. It's a brilliant use for the fruity pink wine and a fun way to show off the flavour of sweet strawberries on hot summer days, especially when you have a few guests. When you want to skip the wine, a light juice will do just fine! Scan the supermarket aisles for white grape or cranberry juice. The grape juice is easier to find, though the cranberry version is around. Either fruit complements the frozen strawberry blend wonderfully, so go with what you can find! You can make a good Frosé with the more common, red-coloured cranberry juice, though the flavour profile of the white version is softer and mimics the wine in this drink a bit better.

Serves 4

350ml white grape, white cranberry, or red cranberry juice, chilled
280g sliced, frozen strawberries
10 ice cubes, or as needed
15ml Simple Syrup (see page 13), or 2 tbsp granulated sugar, or to taste
2 tbsp freshly-squeezed lemon juice, or to taste
1 fresh whole or sliced strawberry per glass, to garnish

Add the juice, frozen strawberries, ice cubes, Simple Syrup and lemon juice to a blender. Blend well, taste, then add more syrup (or sugar) and lemon juice to taste. Pour into frozen glasses (store excess in the fridge for up to 2 days), and garnish with the fresh strawberries.

VARIATIONS

If you have access to one, use a non-alcoholic rosé instead of the juice. Since traditional wine naturally produces alcohol, you'll often see these labelled as 'alcohol-removed' wines. Have fun adding other fruits to the blender – watermelon, mango, papaya or whatever is available! Cut it up and add a twist to the Frosé. If you have it, a splash of sparkling or soda water is a great addition, too.

CRANBERRY–BASIL SANGRIA

Sangria typically includes wine – white or red – but this fruity drink doesn't require it. In non-alcoholic versions, fruit juice does the trick. It's a great jug drink to serve up to a few friends, incredibly easy, and the flavour possibilities are limited only by your imagination. To get you started, I offer the Cranberry-basil Sangria. Basil is one of the easiest herbs to grow in a garden – and, in many climates, the basil harvest tends to coincide with cranberry and apple season. You can use a non-alcoholic wine to enhance this recipe – however, this particular recipe relies on readily available bottles of cranberry juice. You can use either fresh or frozen cranberries, but be sure to use fresh basil, and feel free to play with the many varieties of flavoured sparkling waters available.

Serves 4

710ml cranberry juice (white or red as a wine substitute)
120ml freshly squeezed orange juice
2 tbsp sugar
1 orange, sliced
1 apple, cored and sliced
100g cranberries, fresh or frozen
10g (packed) basil leaves
350ml sparkling water
ice cubes
3–5 cranberries, 1 orange slice and 1 sprig of fresh basil per glass

Combine the cranberry juice, orange juice and sugar in a jug, and stir until the sugar dissolves. Add the orange slices, apple slices and cranberries. Cover, and place in the fridge overnight. When ready to serve, pour the sangria into ice-filled glasses, top with sparkling water and garnish with cranberries, basil and orange slices.

TIP

When you find fresh cranberries in the autumn, freeze them for later use; they make great ice cube substitutes and will thaw as the sangria rests overnight.

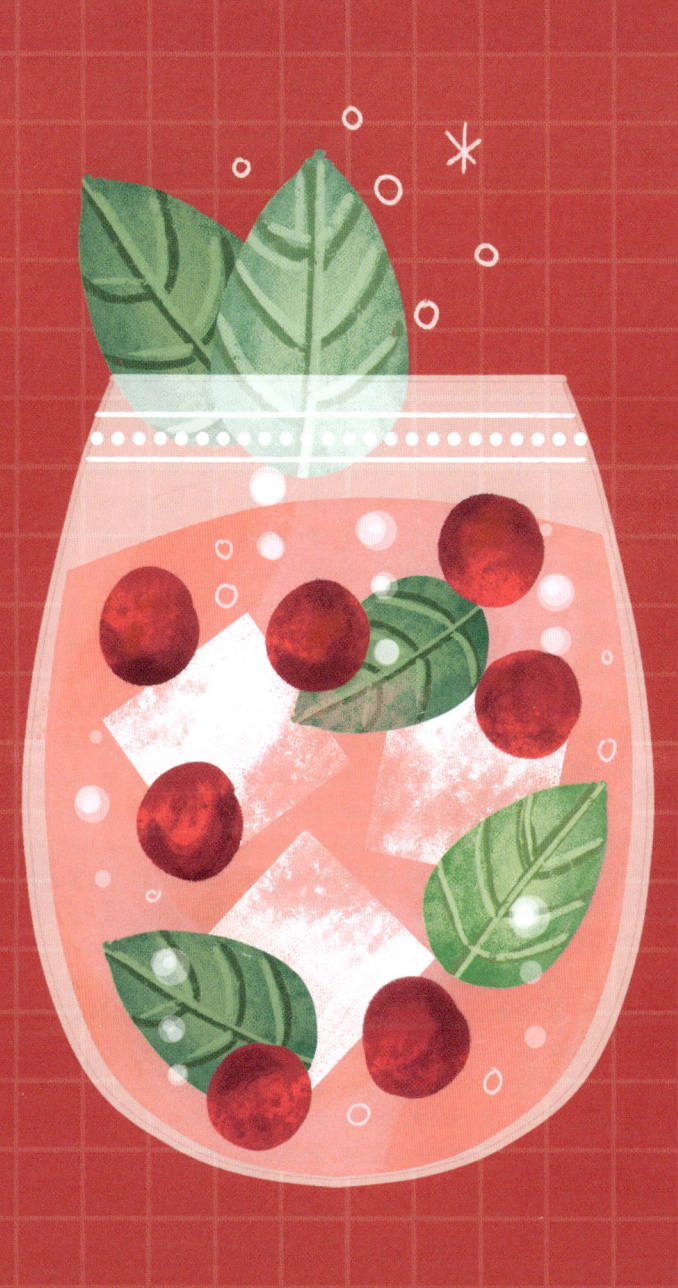

PALOMITA

Featuring the piquant taste of grapefruit in a sparkling highball, the Paloma is a fabulous drink that perfectly encapsulates the Spanish word for 'dove' that it is named after. The Palomita is a popular rendition that typically swaps the tequila for vodka. So, in this free-spirited take, a light zero-proof gin or non-alcoholic botanical spirit is a good choice. Look out for one with a fruity, floral flavour profile (often labelled as a 'botanical spirit'), rather than those that feature the juniper and spices of a traditional gin replica, as these don't work particularly well against grapefruit. With your base spirit of choice, you can then choose to use grapefruit juice with soda water or sparkling water, or alongside a grapefruit-flavoured fizzy drink. The juice offers the most pronounced citrus flavour, while grapefruit-flavoured carbonated drinks are the sweetest. In this recipe, I opt for the former because the drink's sweetness is controllable and not reliant on a fizzy drink.

Serves 1

60ml floral non-alcoholic
  botanical spirit
15ml freshly-squeezed
  lime juice
90ml freshly-squeezed
  grapefruit juice
15ml Rosemary Syrup
  (see page 15), or to taste
soda water, sparkling water
  or a grapefruit-flavoured
  fizzy drink, to top
ice cubes
1 lime wedge or grapefruit
  half-moon, to garnish

Into a highball glass filled with the ice, pour the spirit, lime and grapefruit juices, plus the syrup. Stir well, then top with soda water. Garnish with the lime wedge or grapefruit half-moon.

VARIATION

If you have a zero-proof tequila, try it in this recipe! Vanilla Simple Syrup is a great alternative to Rosemary Syrup, and it complements the grapefruit. Cut a vanilla pod into pieces and leave it to infuse in the standard Simple Syrup recipe (see page 13) as it cools, then strain out the vanilla and bottle the syrup.

SMOKY SOUR

A little smoke, a little sweetness and a little sour – the Smoky Sour is a boldly-flavoured mocktail that's fun to construct. You even get to light something on fire! It's a take on the classic Whisky Sour, using a non-alcoholic whisky and pairing it with lemon juice and a special syrup. The egg white is entirely optional, though it does add a luscious foam top to the cocktail. And, if you have a fresh sprig of rosemary on hand, you can smoke the glass before pouring the drink for another layer of flavour. The syrup is flavoured with cinnamon and lapsang souchong tea, which is pine-smoked, and that flavour adds an interesting aspect that could be likened to a smoky whisky. However, since it is potent, you'll want to remove the tea before the cinnamon to ensure a decent balance of flavours.

Serves 1

fresh rosemary sprig,
   about 5cm long
60ml zero-proof whisky
20ml freshly-squeezed
   lemon juice
20ml Cinnamon-lapsang
   Souchong Tea Syrup
   (see page 17)
1 egg white (optional)
ice cubes
1 lemon twist, to garnish

Light the rosemary sprig on fire using a long match, and let it burn (this may be best done over the sink or other water source for safety purposes). Extinguish the flame by blowing out the fire, then place it in an old-fashioned glass while still smoking. Meanwhile, pour the other ingredients into a cocktail shaker, and dry shake (without ice). Fill the shaker with the ice and shake again for at least 30 seconds. Remove the rosemary (if you prefer) and strain the cocktail into the glass. Garnish with the lemon twist.

VARIATION

Try this one with a zero-proof tequila.

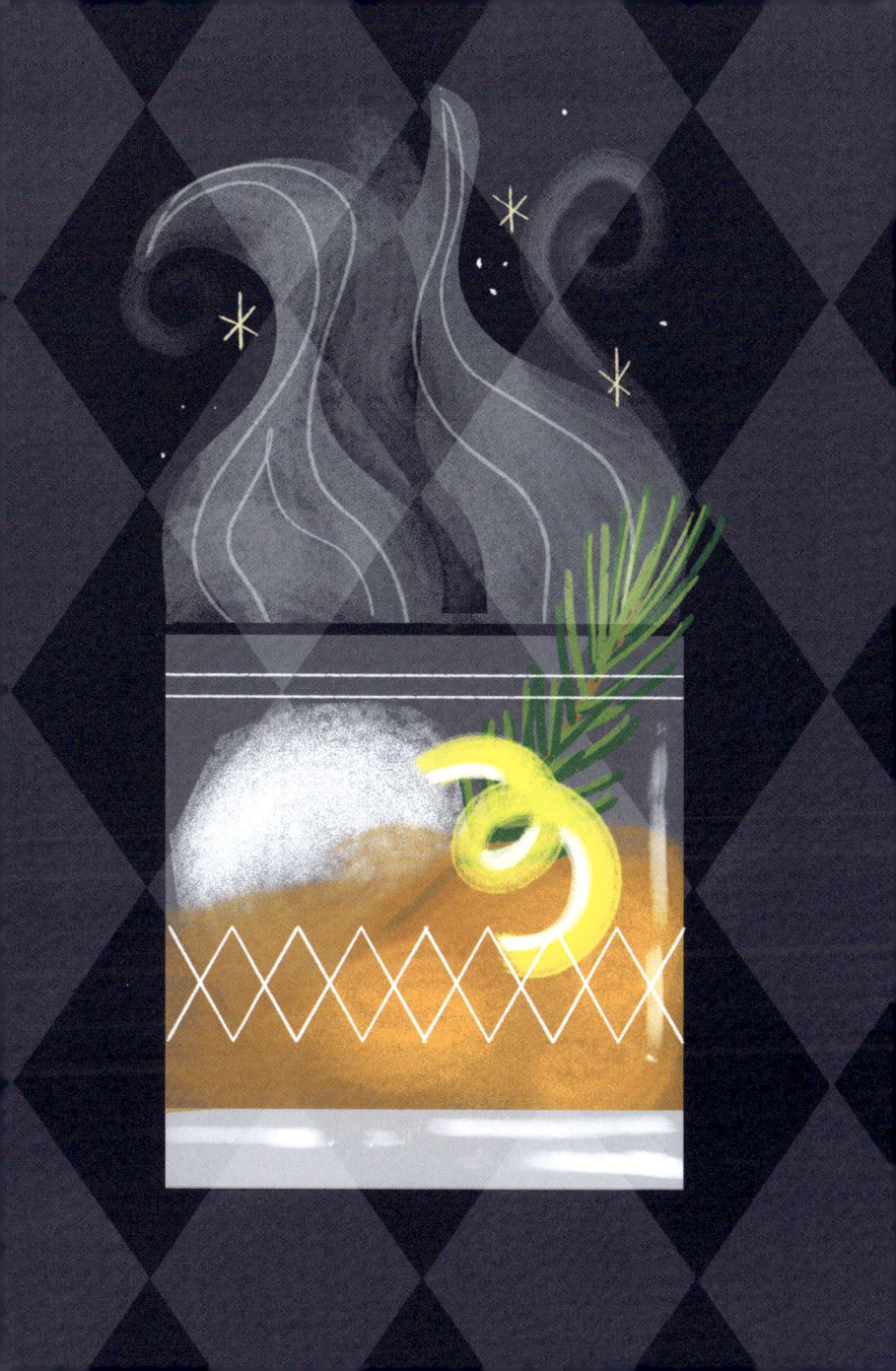

NO-APEROL SPRITZ

Some cocktails rely on a branded liquor. Recreating them without those products can be a challenge; with this in mind, I will occasionally recommend brand-name ingredients that may help you to achieve the best possible results – though I encourage you to explore the market as it evolves, because you might find some fantastic newbies pop up that are equally enjoyable. The No-groni (see page 56) and the No-Aperol Spritz are perfect examples: both, in their original guises, rely on a specific aperitif that is uniquely formulated and gives each cocktail its signature flavour. In the Aperol Spritz, it's the bitter-sweet Italian liquor (you guessed it!) Aperol. When seeking out a non-alcoholic alternative, you want something with a dominant bitter orange profile, backed by an array of interesting botanicals. With the rise of sober curious drinkers, it's an endeavour several companies strive for, and Lyre's Non-alcoholic Italian Orange Aperitivo is one of the leaders in this ultra-specific realm. To complete the No-Aperol Spritz, Prosecco is replaced with tonic water because it has a dry profile similar to the Italian sparkling wine. If you want more sparkle without tonic's bitterness, a splash of soda water evens it out nicely. A few orange slices are absolutely necessary, as they bring the flavours of this drink into balance.

Serves 1

1–2 orange slices
   (full wheels or halves)
ice cubes
60ml non-alcoholic bitter
   orange aperitivo, such as
   Lyre's (see headnote)
60ml tonic water
30ml soda water or
   sparkling water
   (optional)

Fill a highball glass or large wine glass with the ice, adding at least one orange slice amongst the icy filling. Pour in the orange aperitif, then the tonic water, and top it off with soda water, if you're using some.

NO–GRONI

The Negroni relies on Campari – there are no debates about that in the cocktail world. The crimson, bitter Italian aperitif is simply not replicable, because it's a proprietary recipe that's been around since 1860. In the Negroni, it is paired with gin and sweet vermouth, so you can imagine that transforming this alcohol-only cocktail into a spirit-free beverage is a challenge. Fortunately, the zero-proof spirit makers of the world have been on it since the very beginning. For a great No-groni, pick up a juniper-forward, zero-proof gin that replicates a London dry style. You'll also want to grab a non-alcoholic sweet vermouth. And, for that elusive Campari substitute, there are a few interesting choices. Like the No-Aperol Spritz (see page 55), look for bitter-sweet orange aperitivo options – Lyre's has a great one (along with a sweet vermouth alternative). Ghia aperitif, which includes gentian root (the main bitter ingredient in Campari), also works really well in this drink. With a trio of non-alcoholic substitutes, whose flavour will vary greatly as you explore brands, be sure to adapt the No-groni recipe to every new combination. The equal measurements are only a suggestion and starting point – pour, stir, taste and add more of something to find your balance.

Serves 1

30ml zero-proof gin
   or non-alcoholic
   botanical spirit
30ml non-alcoholic sweet
   vermouth
30ml non-alcoholic bitter
   orange aperitivo, such
   as Lyre's
2 dashes orange bitters
2 dashes aromatic bitters
ice cubes
1 orange twist, to garnish

Pour the ingredients into a cocktail shaker filled with the ice, and stir very well. Strain into a chilled old-fashioned glass over ice cubes and garnish with the orange twist.

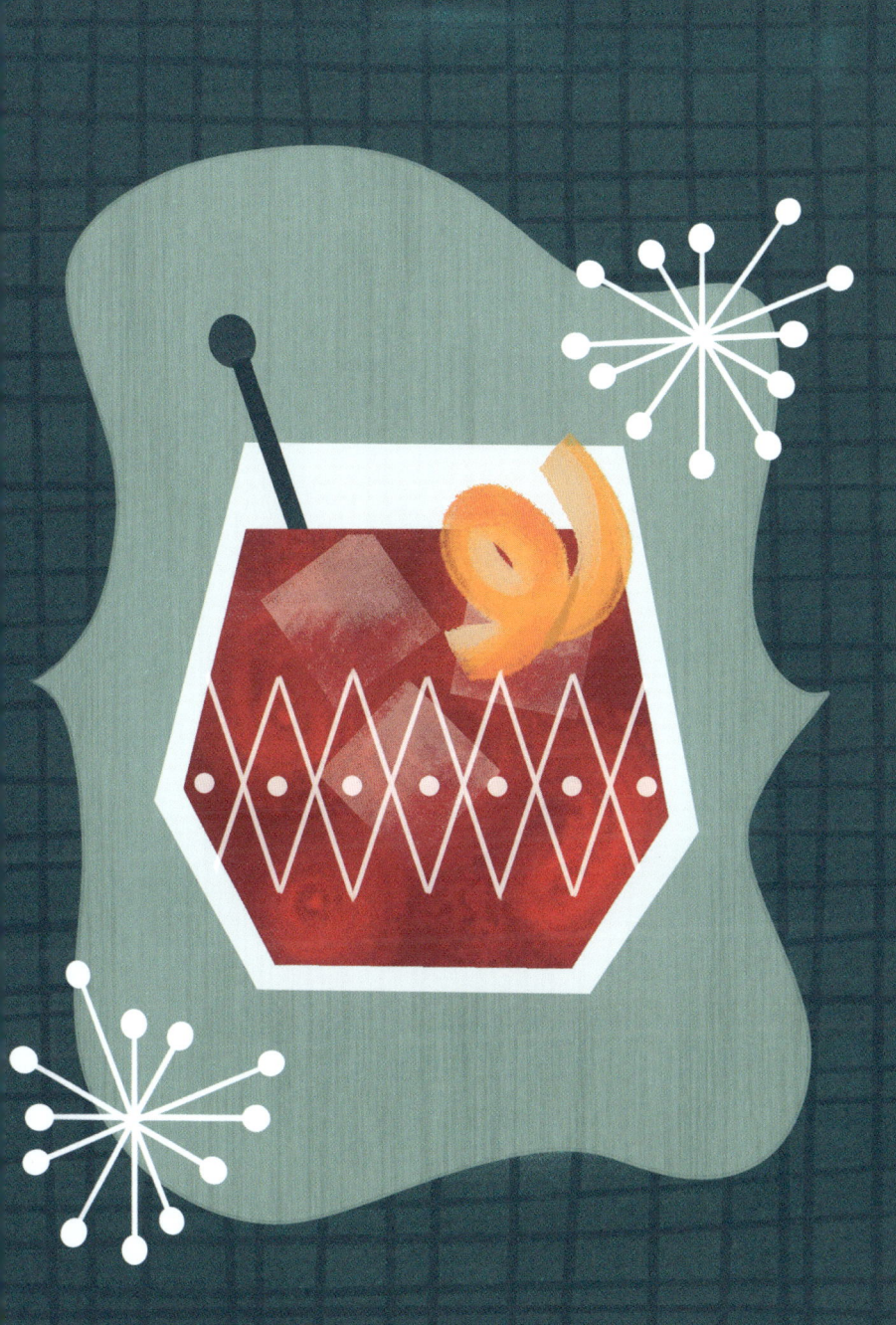

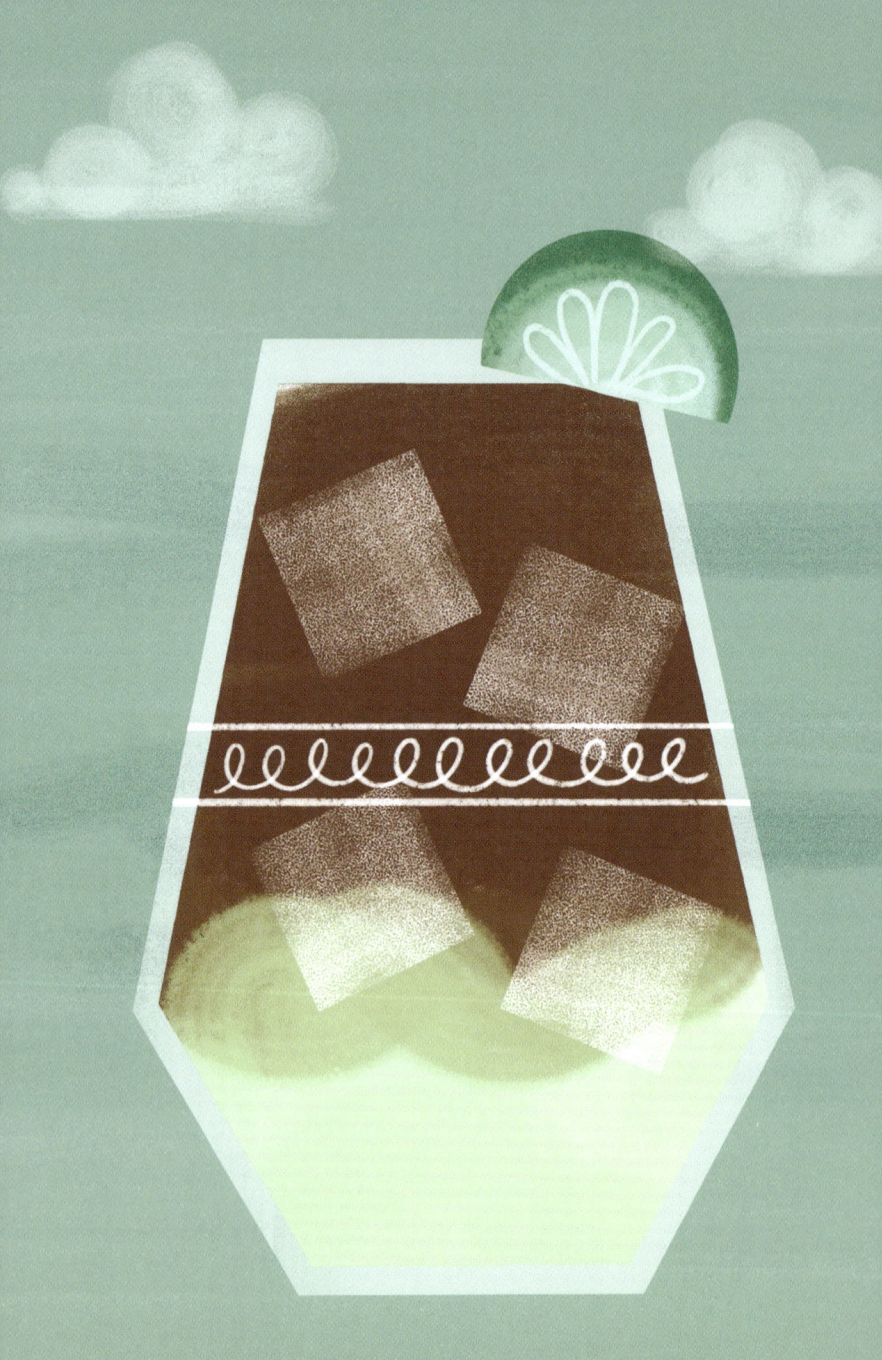

DARK 'N' BLUSTERY

Based on a rum highball, which is really nothing more than rum and ginger beer, the Dark 'n' Blustery is a snappy mocktail. It's one of those year-round beverages that will pick you up, enliven your senses and is as great after a long day at work as it is with dinner. The Dark 'n' Stormy cocktail is traditionally made with Goslings Black Seal Rum, which is rich and dark, and the perfect pairing for a spicy ginger beer (Barritt's is the apparent 'original' brand of choice, but try Homemade Ginger Beer, see page 86). In a non-alcoholic take on that, you'll want some additional sweetener. Since zero-proof rums are not as sweet, a touch of Simple Syrup makes up the difference. This should also be adjusted to the ginger beer because some are very sweet. Also, seek out darker zero-proof rums (sometimes called 'cane spirits', meaning they're derived from cane sugar) here – if they're amber-coloured, great; any that are clear may be okay, but will not create the ideal Dark 'n' Blustery.

Serves 1

ice cubes
15ml Simple Syrup
  (see page 13)
20ml freshly-squeezed
  lime juice
60ml zero-proof dark rum
60–90ml ginger beer
1 lime wedge, to garnish

Into a highball glass filled with the ice, pour the Simple Syrup, lime juice and zero-proof rum. Stir well, then top with ginger beer and garnish with the lime wedge.

BUZZY BEE'S KNEES

If you know anything about the early twentieth century, you'll recognize the slang, 'that's the bee's knees'. The original gin cocktail came out of those days. It was created by Frank Meier, who was a bartender at the Hotel Ritz in Paris during the 1920s. Really, that phrase describes the cocktail wonderfully, and it's one of the easiest you can mix up. Essentially a sweeter version of the Gin Sour, this cocktail requires gin, Honey Syrup and lemon juice – easy peasy! Transforming it into a mocktail is just as easy: choose a zero-proof gin or non-alcoholic botanical spirit, shake it up and you're done. As with the gin choices available today, each non-alcoholic spirit you pour will change the drink's profile completely. It's one that you should use when exploring each new-to-you bottle, because it's such a clean mix with only a hint of sweet and sour, so you can get a real sense of where else that 'spirit' can be used. Beyond freshly-squeezed lemon juice (don't even think about the bottled stuff here), Honey Syrup is essential. After all, it puts the 'bee' in this recipe. (Simple Syrup would suffice, but it just doesn't have the same effect.) Besides, the story of the cocktail's creation is that honey took the edge off some of the less-than-desirable bath-tub gins of Prohibition, so if you're easing into the taste of gin substitutes, it's a natural place to begin training your palate.

Serves 1

ice cubes
60ml zero-proof gin
   or non-alcoholic
   botanical spirit
20ml Honey Syrup
   (see page 14) or Simple
   Syrup (see page 13;
   see headnote)
15ml freshly-squeezed
   lemon juice

Into a cocktail shaker filled with the ice, add the ingredients. Shake well, then strain into a chilled cocktail glass.

VARIATIONS

Play with flavoured Honey Syrups to give the drink a fun twist. Lavender-honey (see page 14) is a fun option, as is Rosemary (see page 15).

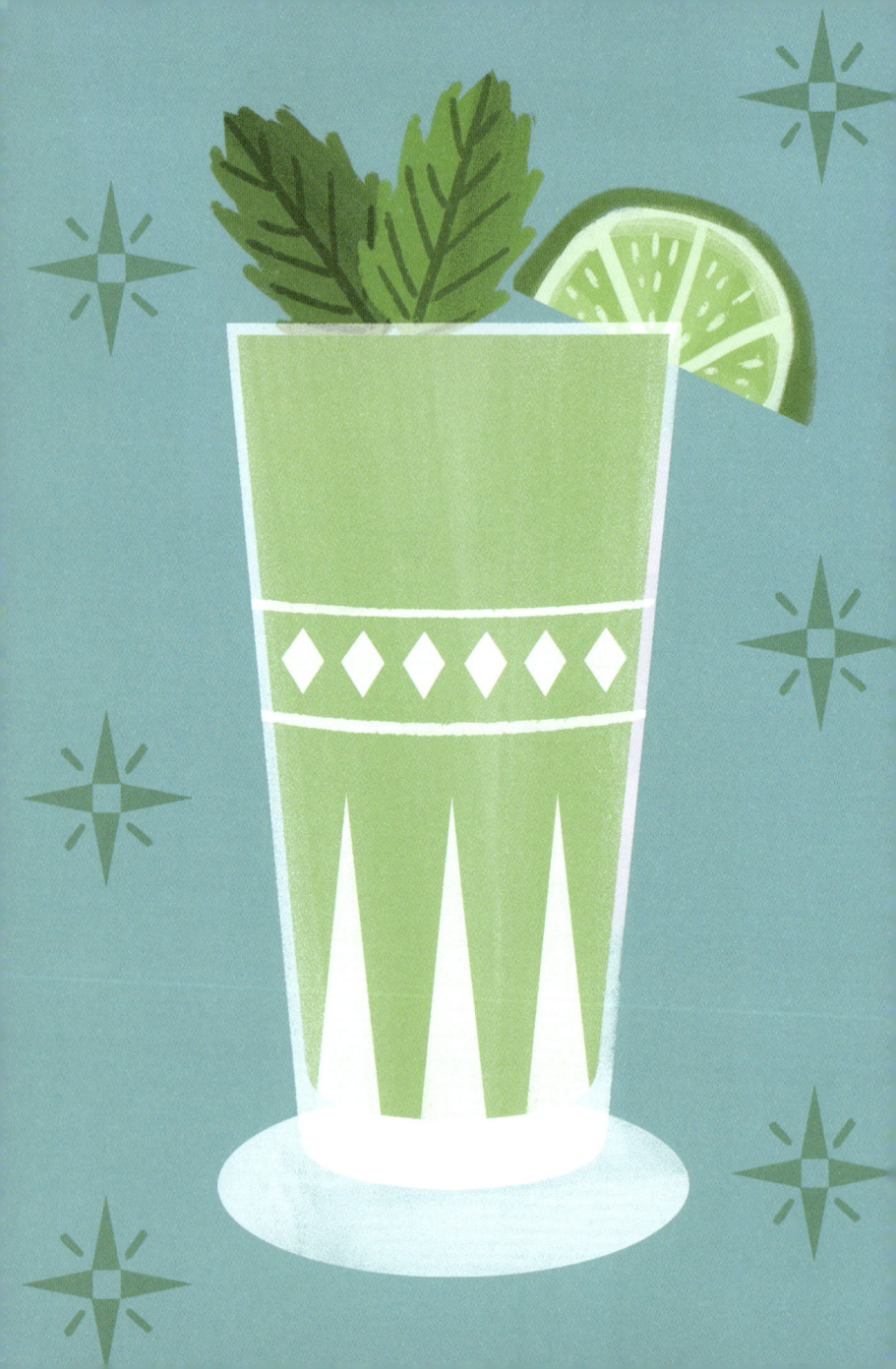

MATCHA MOJITO

Matcha is an interesting green tea that's sold as a fine powder. It has an intriguing umami flavour with a noticeable vegetal tone, and it pairs surprisingly well with the classic mojito ingredients of lime and mint. There are two grades of matcha available. Culinary matcha is best reserved for foods and beverages with heavier ingredients, like lattes. Ceremonial matcha is perfect for any drink, and the preferred choice for this mojito. Since the matcha is a powder, it doesn't steep like tea leaves do. Instead, you'll want to sift it through a fine-mesh sieve, then mix it with warm water until it dissolves (traditionally, this is done with a bamboo whisk, called a chasen, though a small kitchen whisk works, too). Let the tea cool for a few minutes, then you're ready to build the drink. While rum is typically included in a mojito, I have yet to find a zero-proof rum that I truly enjoy in a Matcha Mojito. Give a few a try, though, or go with a zero-proof gin or non-alcoholic botanical spirit.

Serves 1

1 tsp matcha, sifted
60ml filtered or distilled
  hot water
60ml zero-proof gin or
  rum, or non-alcoholic
  botanical spirit
30ml freshly-squeezed
  lime juice
30ml Simple Syrup
  (see page 13)
5–6 fresh mint leaves,
  torn
ice cubes
60–90ml sparkling or
  soda water, or to taste
1 lime slice and fresh mint
  sprig, to garnish

Add the sifted matcha to a small bowl with the hot water, and whisk until dissolved and lump free. Let cool, then pour into a highball glass. Add the spirit (if using), lime, syrup and mint leaves. Muddle well to release the lime juice and mint essence. Fill the glass with ice and top with sparkling or soda water, then garnish with the lime slice and mint sprig.

SOBER SIDECAR

An iconic classic, the Sidecar is certainly not a light drink. It's spirit-heavy, featuring brandy or bourbon with triple sec, but once you find a suitable balance of sweet and sour, it is a thing of beauty. As with many cocktails, transforming it into a free-spirited drink requires experimentation. In the Sober Sidecar, I recommend exploring your zero-proof whisky options first. For more of a brandy-like mouth-feel, give some of the red-coloured aperitif options a try. I honestly find these to be more pleasant than the bolder whiskies, but also enjoy splitting the two equally. Whichever base you pour, remember that the triple sec and lemon should be adapted each time. Take notes, and all will be well for the next round!

Serves 1

ice cubes
60ml zero-proof whisky
   or red-coloured aperitif
30ml non-alcoholic triple
   sec, or Orange Syrup
   (see page 16)
20ml freshly-squeezed
   lemon juice
1 lemon peel, to garnish

Into a cocktail shaker filled with the ice, add the liquids and shake well. Strain into a chilled cocktail glass, then garnish with the lemon peel.

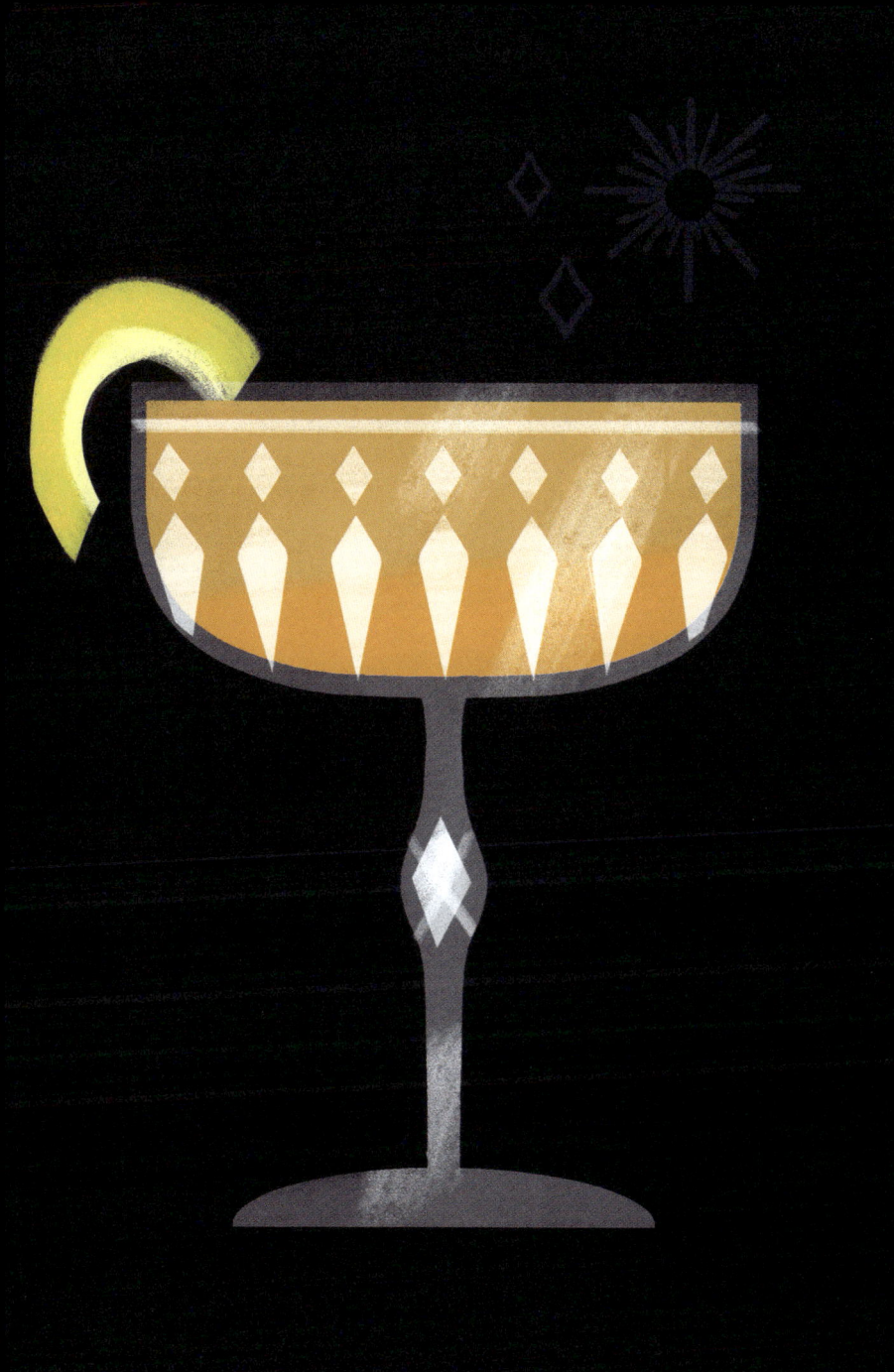

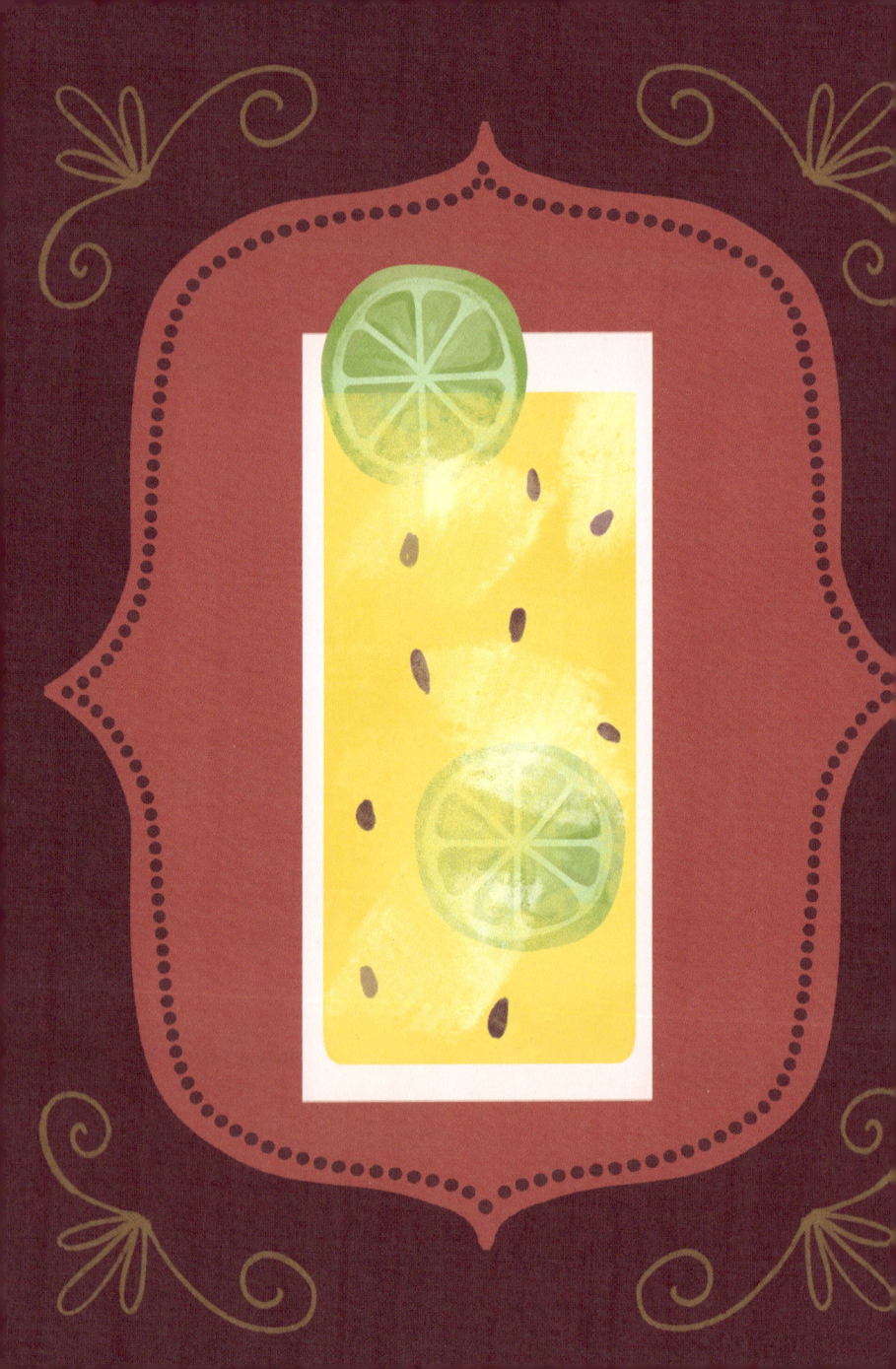

PASSION FRUIT FIZZ

The passion fruit is one of those beautiful exotic fruits that deserves more of a spotlight in drinks. Its sweet taste is a perfect base for a tall, sparkling beverage. Make it with one of the non-alcoholic spirits residing in your drinks cabinet; gin, rum or tequila – all three work well. Passion fruit happens to be an excellent match for ginger syrup – try it, and you'll likely be pleasantly surprised! If you have access to fresh passion fruit, purée the flesh in a blender. You can strain out the pulp if you like, but it's not necessary, and those tiny black seeds look stunning in the glass. No fresh passion fruit available? Pick up some bottled passion fruit juice to use instead.

Serves 1

ice cubes
60ml zero-proof gin or non-alcoholic botanical spirit, rum or tequila
60ml fresh passion fruit purée or bottled passion fruit juice (see headnote)
30ml ginger-infused Simple Syrup (for recipe, see Home-made Ginger Beer, page 86)
30ml freshly-squeezed lime juice
120–180ml soda water or sparkling water
1 lime slice, to garnish

In a cocktail shaker filled with the ice, pour the spirit, passion fruit, ginger syrup and lime juice. Shake vigorously, then strain over fresh ice in a tall glass. Top with club soda and garnish with the lime slice.

VARIATIONS

Use unflavoured Simple Syrup (see page 13) or try this one with a non-alcoholic triple sec (see page 18). This drink also works with the egg white of a classic fizz cocktail; remember to dry shake the ingredients, then add ice and shake again (see page 82, for mixing tips).

NON-ALCOHOLIC FRENCH 75

Tall and sparkling, with a lovely lemon flavour, just try to resist the French 75! Taking this one into the free-spirited world is actually not too difficult: simply swap the gin for a non-alcoholic botanical spirit, and the champagne for a non-alcoholic sparkling wine. It's a brilliant celebratory drink that pairs wonderfully with nearly any dinner. As with many of these mocktails, your experience of a Non-alcoholic French 75 will vary depending on the alternative ingredients you decide to choose. Try it with a juniper-forward, zero-proof gin, or one that's on the lighter, more floral side. There are several non-alcoholic sparkling wines on the market now; you can also use sparkling grape juice, cider, soda water or tonic water. What I really like about the clean taste of this cocktail is that you can add a subtle twist using flavoured syrups. The floral options such as lavender, rosemary and elderflower are simply fantastic. For a fruitier French 75, make strawberry syrup; or, in mid-summer, give it a watermelon, honeydew or cantaloupe twist. The base is here – your imagination can then decide where to take it next!

Serves 1

60ml zero-proof gin or non-alcoholic botanical spirit, chilled
15ml Simple Syrup (see page 13), flavoured or plain
15ml freshly-squeezed lemon juice
120ml non-alcoholic sparkling wine, grape juice, cider, or sparkling or soda water, chilled
1 lemon twist, to garnish

Pour the spirit, syrup and lemon juice into a champagne flute. Top with the sparkling beverage of your choice, then drape the long lemon twist over the rim.

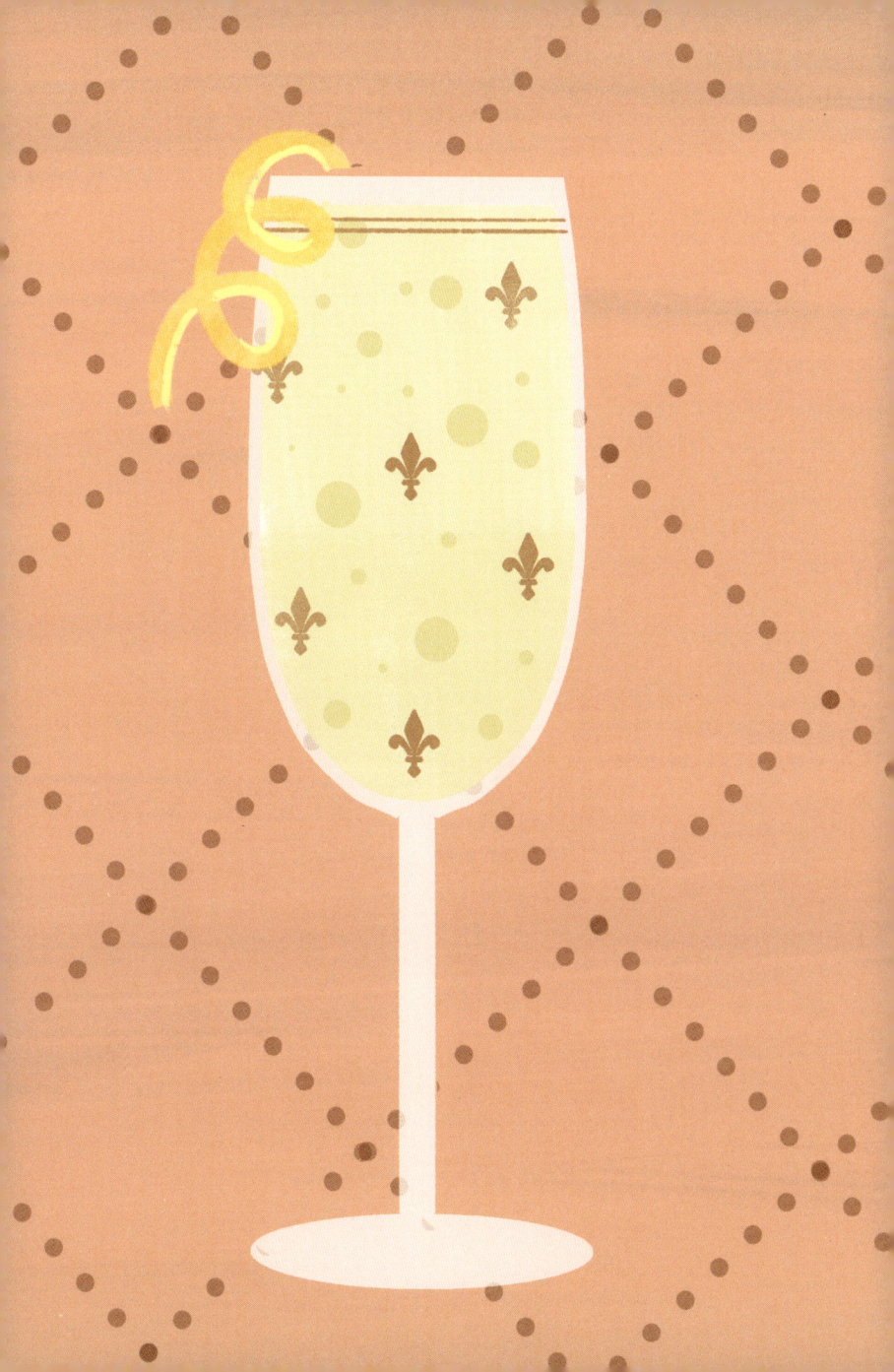

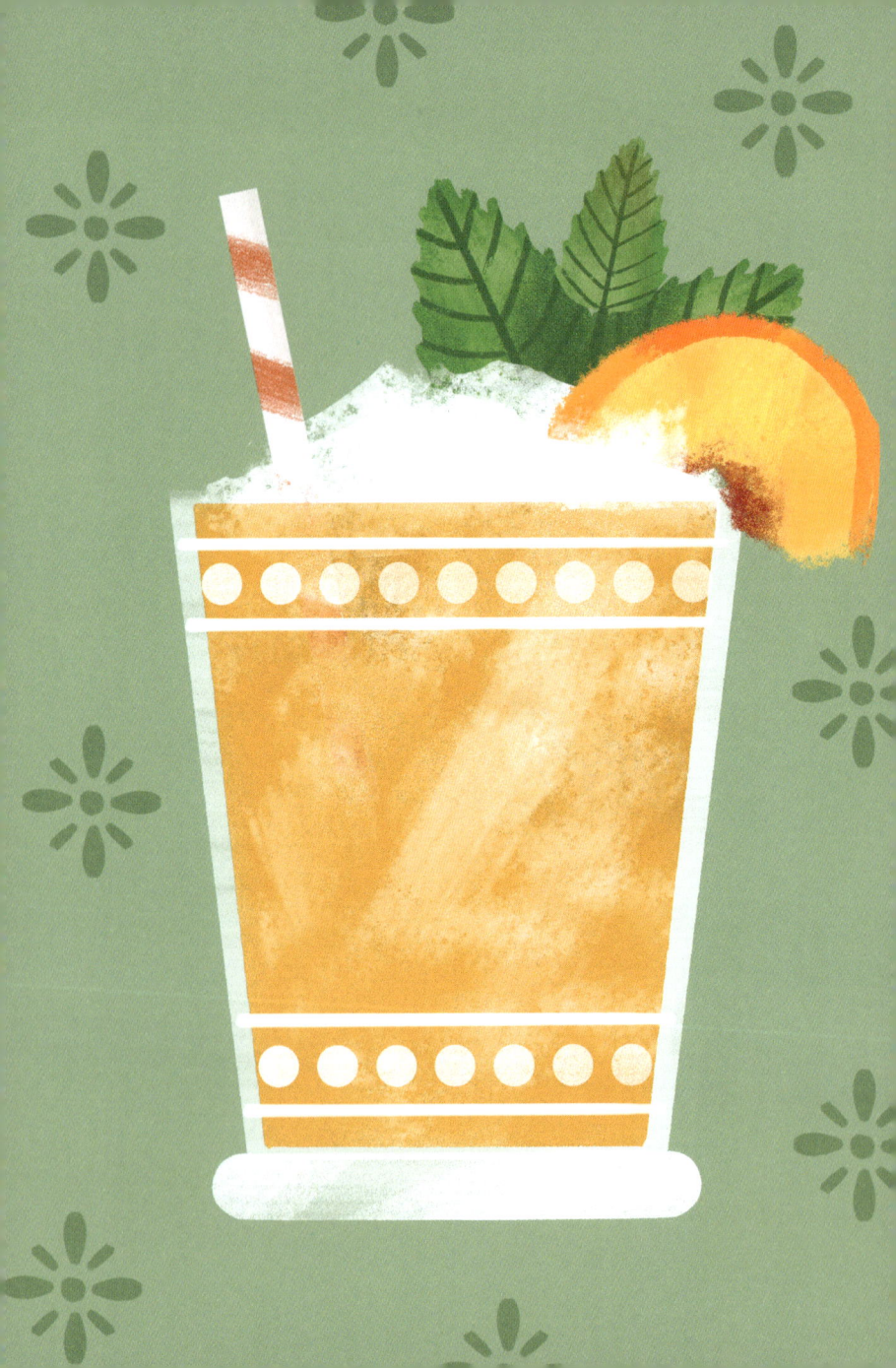

GRAND DERBY MINT JULEP

Bourbon, bourbon, bourbon. . . the one true requirement for a great Mint Julep. (OK, there's mint, too!) So, what do you do when avoiding a shot of Kentucky's finest liquor? Switch to a zero-proof bourbon and downplay the spicy edge with a bit more syrup and a couple of peach slices. This Grand Derby Mint Julep is a very simple take on the classic julep recipe. Fresh mint is muddled with Simple Syrup, the 'bourbon' is stirred in, the glass is filled with crushed ice, then it's stirred until the glass is ultra-frosty (don't skimp on this step – the dilution you get from stirring is key). Better yet, build it in a copper or tin julep cup – they get frostier than glass and are the traditional choice. Fresh mint is preferred, and if you have a bounty in the garden or kitchen, preserve it by making a mint-flavoured Simple Syrup (see pages 12–13).

Serves 1

2 mint sprigs, torn
  leaves only
15ml Simple Syrup
  (see page 13)
½ white peach or
  1 apricot, sliced
65ml zero-proof
  bourbon
ice cubes
1 mint sprig and peach
  slice, to garnish

In the bottom of a double old-fashioned glass (or copper or tin tumbler), add mint leaves, syrup and peach slices. Muddle well. Add the zero-proof bourbon; fill the glass with ice. Stir well until the glass is covered with frost; garnish with the mint sprig and peach slice.

VARIATION

Try the julep with a zero-proof gin or non-alcoholic botanical spirit of any variety. Many people enjoy a gin julep more than the whisky version. Use raw (e.g. demerara) or brown sugar in the Simple Syrup for a richer flavour. Honey (see page 14) is a nice alternative in this recipe, too.

SPARKLING PEACH SUNRISE

If you are smitten by the Sweet Sunrise (see page 32) and Bellini Sparkler (see page 28), you're sure to fall for the Sparkling Peach Sunrise. A recipe I created several years ago, it's a mash-up of those two marvellous mocktails – and just as easy to mix up. In this drink, the base is peach juice, and it's topped with a lemon-lime fizzy drink. (I've also enjoyed it with tonic water.) For that sunrise effect, we employ grenadine, which also adds a sweetness that will tempt you into taking the next sip. It's a great brunch drink, but also a refreshing option for an afternoon on the patio or an accompaniment to dinner.

Serves 1

ice cubes
60ml peach juice
120–150ml lemon-lime
 carbonated drink,
 to taste
20ml grenadine

Fill a tall glass with the ice, pour in the peach juice and top with the fizzy drink, leaving a bit of room at the top. Stir gently, then slowly pour the grenadine into the glass.

VARIATION

As with the Bellini Sparkler, you can swap the peach juice for peach nectar or purée. The latter will create a thicker drink, although the thickness will be offset by the fizzy drink.

RASPBERRY ARNOLD PALMER

One of the most popular booze-free mixed drinks, the Arnold Palmer is little more than lemonade and iced tea. It's cool and refreshing, and adding sweet raspberries enhances this captivating mix, so why not enjoy a fruitier Arnold Palmer? Interestingly enough, for years it became custom to simply pour equal parts of lemonade and iced tea (but that's actually an Arnie Palmer), though the golfing legend enjoyed it with two parts tea and one part lemonade. We're going with his version for the base, because the raspberry muddle adds the perfect amount of sweetness. First, brew 475ml of hot tea, let it cool, then add 1 litre of cold water – this produces the best iced tea flavour without the bitterness or cloudiness of other methods (alternatively, just cold-brew your tea). Second, make some lemonade from scratch (see page 85).

Serves 1

5–6 fresh raspberries
ice cubes
60ml home-made
  lemonade (see page 85),
  chilled
120ml freshly-brewed iced
  tea, chilled (see headnote)
3 fresh raspberries and a
  lemon slice, to garnish

In a tall glass, muddle the raspberries into a thick, juicy pulp. Fill the glass with the ice, then add the lemonade and iced tea. Stir well to combine. Garnish with the raspberries and the lemon slice.

VARIATIONS

I recommend making a raspberry lemonade with a Raspberry Syrup (see page 17), using about 250g of raspberries. Many other fruits would work this way, too, especially strawberries and blueberries. It's also nice with a ginger lemonade (using a ginger-infused syrup – see page 86).

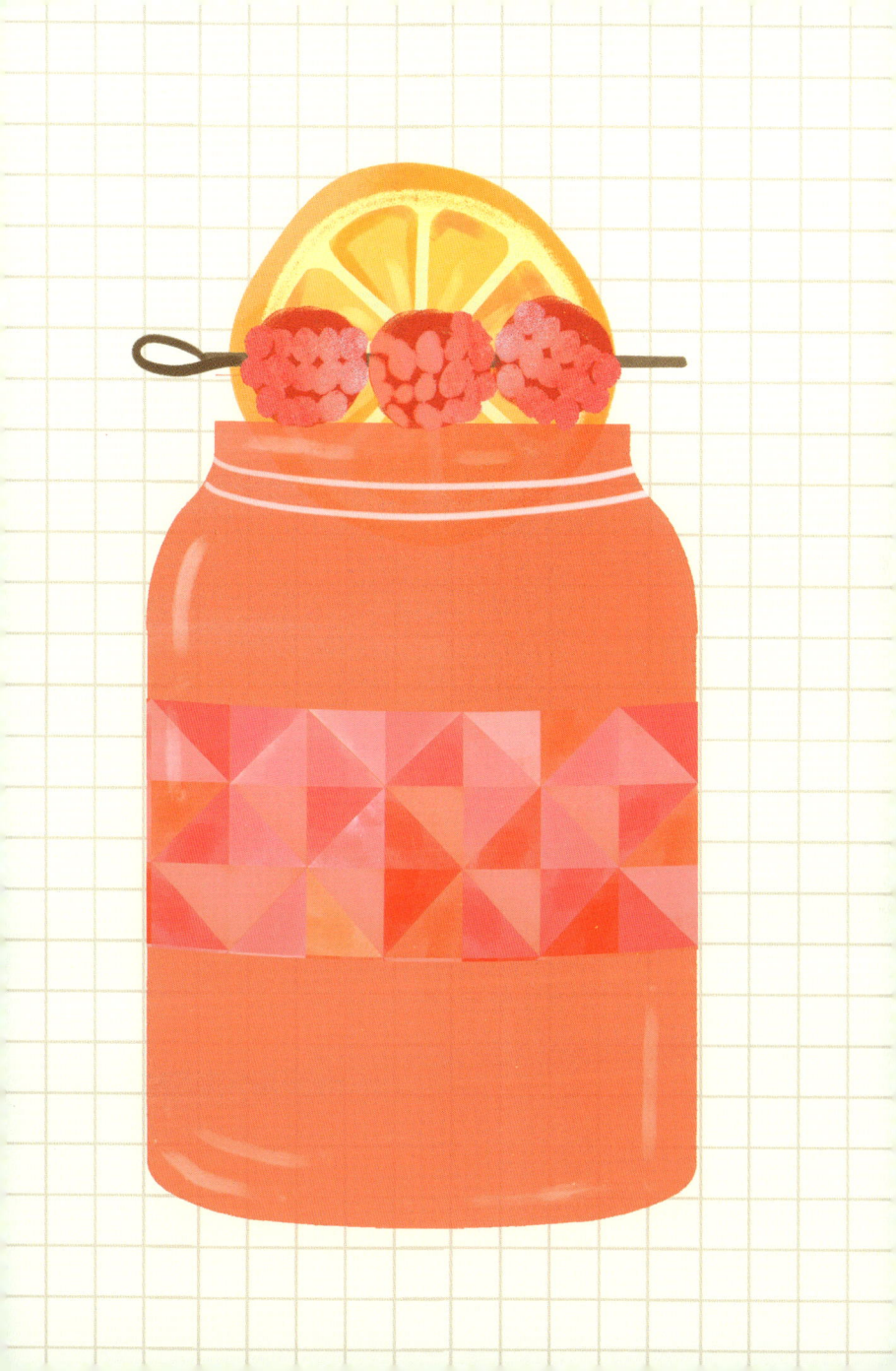

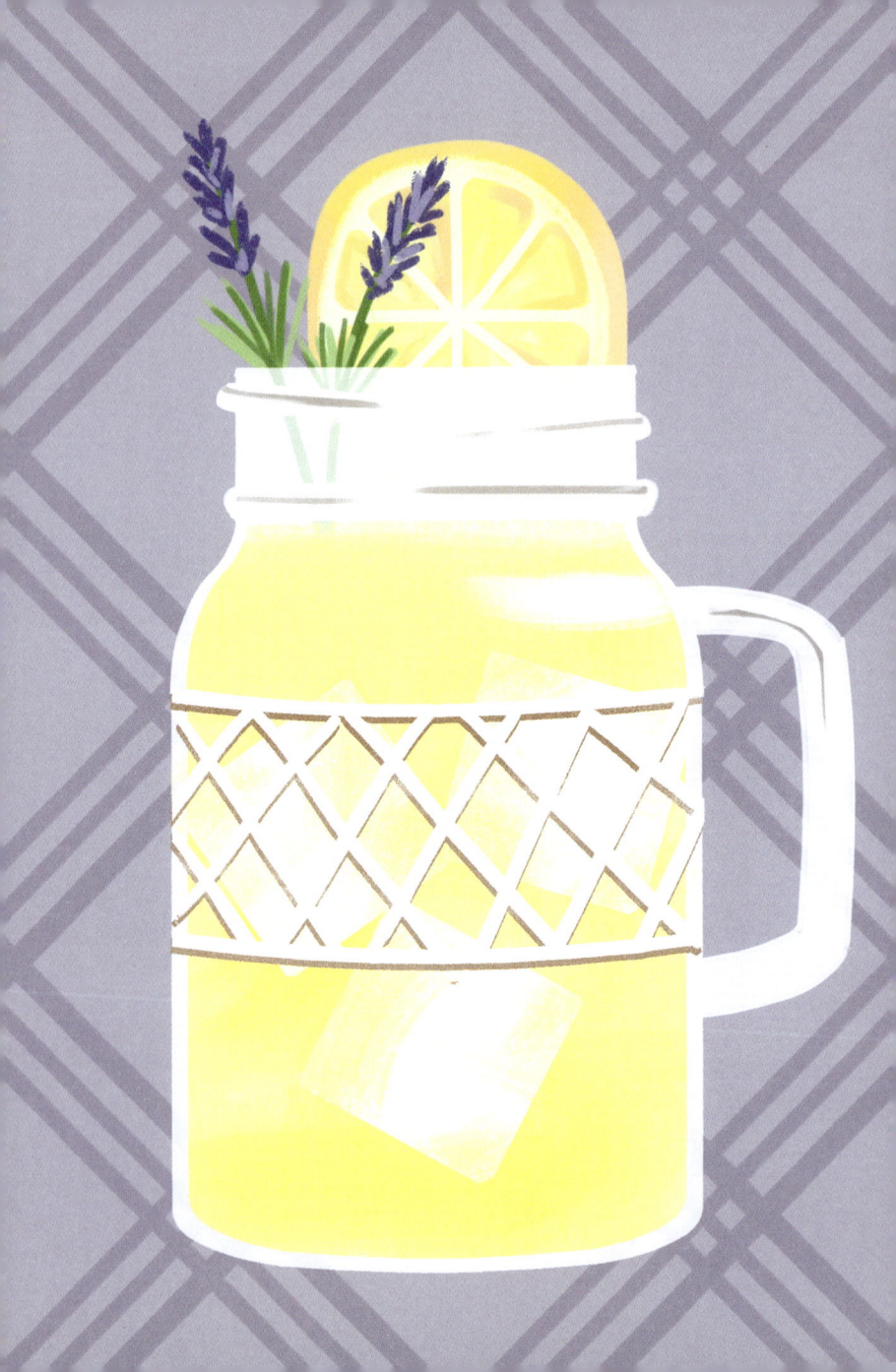

LAVENDER LEMONADE

There's an entire section of my garden dedicated to lavender. Cultivating and harvesting these plants is one of the most pleasant chores I can imagine, and all that lavender deserves to be put to good use. This ingredient appears in many of my drinks, but an all-time favourite is Lavender Lemonade. This recipe makes a full jug, and it's wonderful for entertaining or just stashing in the fridge for a quick summer afternoon refreshment. Like many of my lavender drinks, it begins with a home-made syrup – it really is the best way to get that sweet, floral taste of the tiny purple buds. Rather than an infused Simple Syrup, I have opted for a Lavender-honey Syrup – because a touch of honey adds a nice, rich darkness to the otherwise brightly flavoured mix. A note about lavender: the herb is used for both aromatherapy and culinary purposes. When you intend to use it in food and drinks, make sure it hasn't been sprayed with chemicals. That's easy if you grow it yourself – but when shopping, buy organic lavender to ensure your lavender is safe for consumption. If you cannot lay your hands on fresh lavender sprigs, for your garnish, go with lemon slices alone.

Serves 6–8

350ml freshly-squeezed lemon juice (about 6 fresh lemons)
240–350ml Lavender-honey Syrup (see page 14), to taste
ice cubes, to serve
6–8 lemon slices and fresh lavender sprigs (optional), to garnish

Pour the lemon juice into a large jug, then add 240ml of the Lavender-honey Syrup and 1 litre water. Stir well and taste. Add more syrup to make it sweeter if it's too tart, and more water if it becomes too sweet, stirring and tasting after each addition. It's best to keep the jug chilled, then add the ice to the jug and serving glasses when almost ready to serve (the ice will tame the flavour, so it is best to go a bit strong on the flavour when mixing). Garnish each glass with the lemon slices and fresh lavender sprigs.

SHIRLEY TEMPLE

Before mocktails became a popular alternative for non-drinkers, there were at least three non-alcoholic alternatives you could order at most bars and restaurants: the Raspberry Arnold Palmer (see page 74), Roy Rogers (see page 109) and the sweet, pink-red, sparkling Shirley Temple. Bartenders knew and relied on these drinks when a patron wanted something other than a fizzy drink or water, and the Shirley Temple is surely a favourite among the trio. The secret to a great Shirley Temple? The combination of lemon-lime soda and ginger ale. These two soft drinks are a perfect match, and when you add just a touch of grenadine, you have a wonderful beverage. It is a sweet combination, for sure, as all three ingredients include sugar. So, be sure to add plenty of ice for the necessary chill and dilution, and don't pour in too much grenadine.

Serves 1

ice cubes
½ tbsp grenadine
90ml lemon-lime soda
90ml ginger ale
2–3 fresh or maraschino
  cherries, to garnish

Fill a tall glass with the ice and pour in the grenadine. Fill with equal parts of the two drinks, stir well. Garnish with the cherries.

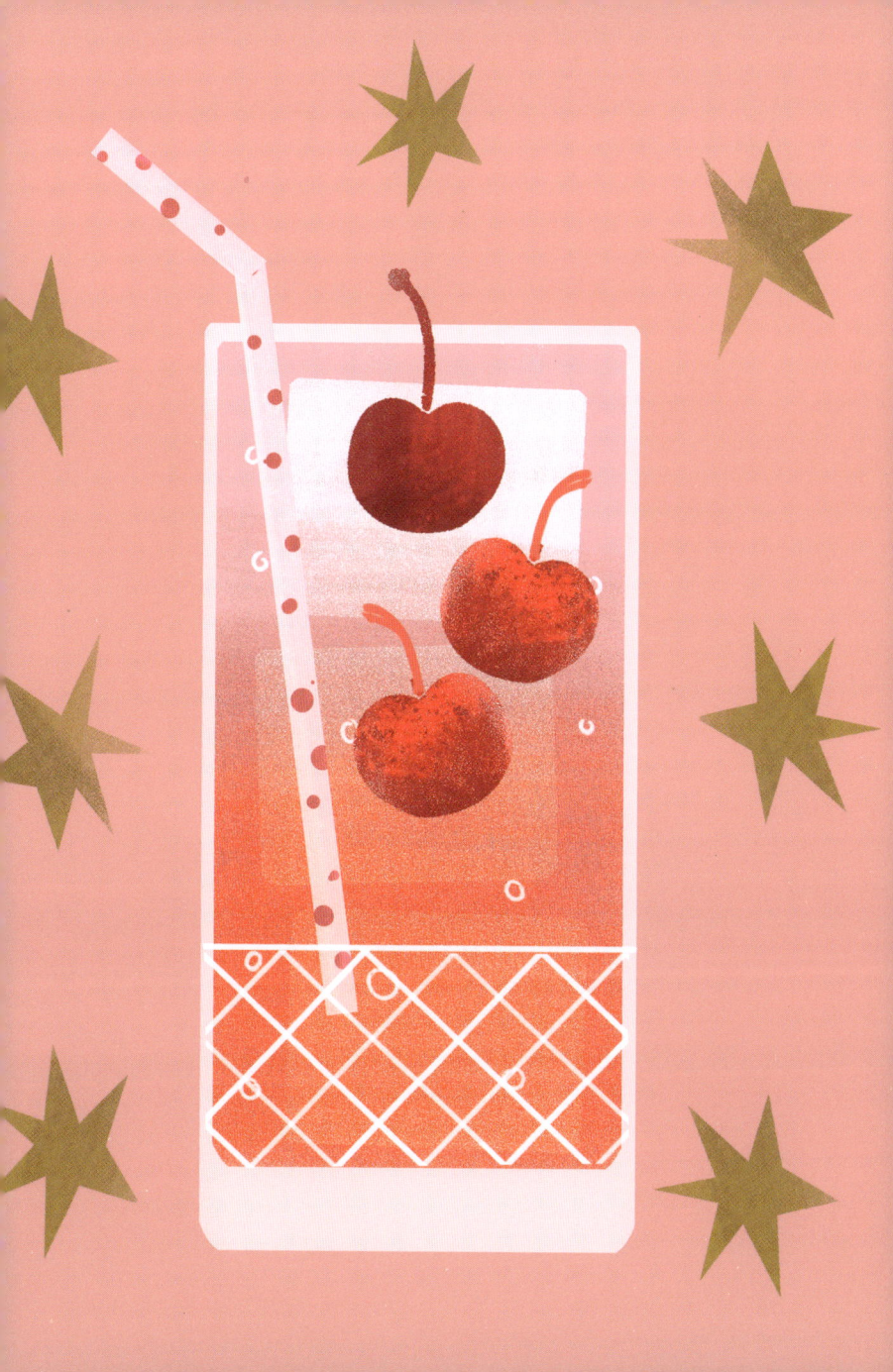

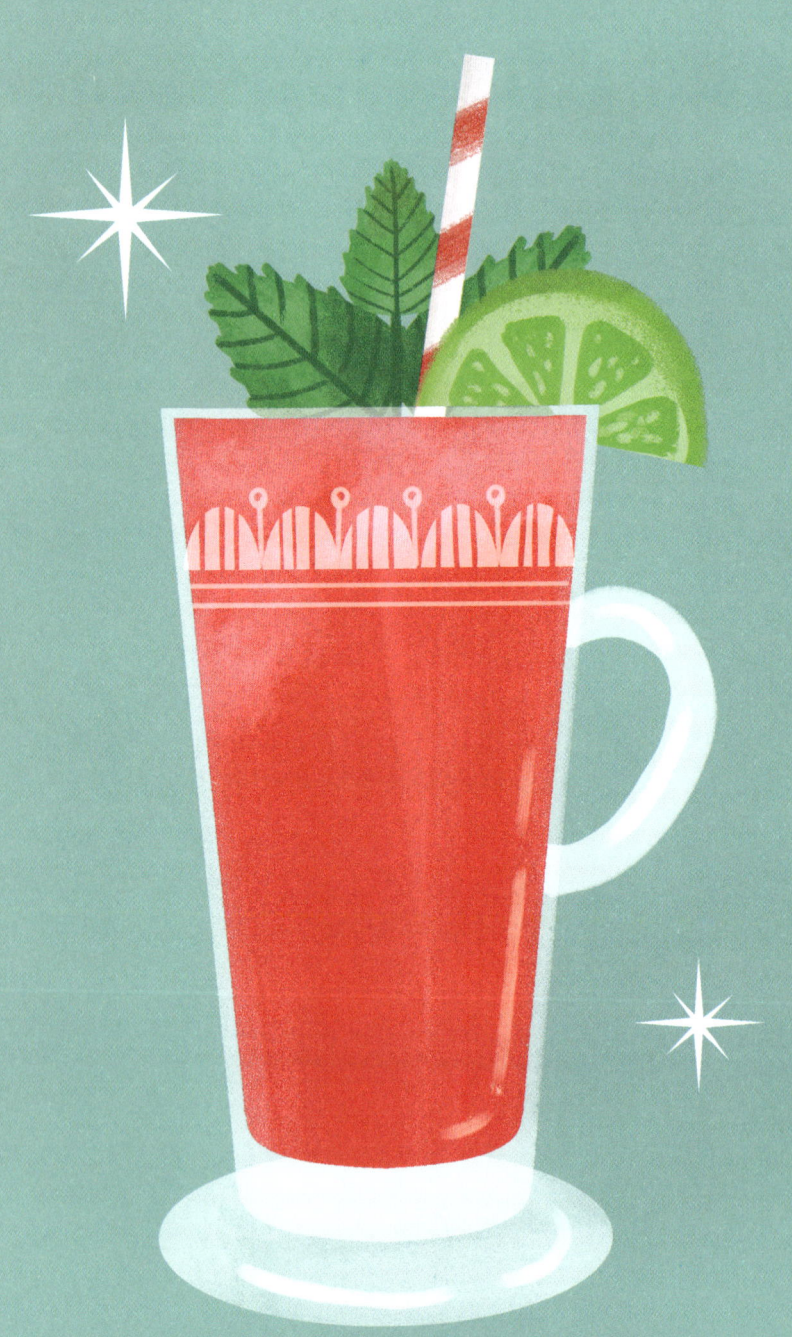

WATERMELON SLUSHIE

A Watermelon Slushie is a real treat on hot summer days. It's a great way to use up excess watermelon from a picnic or barbecue, so you can enjoy an ice-cold slushie later in the week. Strawberries are an ideal pairing with watermelon, though I encourage you to also try tropical fruits such as mango, papaya or pineapple. To accent the entire mix, a handful of fresh basil or mint is a fun addition. For the sweetener, honey is a great option. Simple Syrup or molasses work too; start with just a splash of either – molasses especially – and adjust to taste.

Serves 1

300g frozen watermelon cubes, seedless (or seeds removed before freezing)

35g frozen, chopped strawberries, mango, papaya or pineapple

30ml freshly-squeezed lime juice

1–2 tbsp honey, Simple Syrup (see page 13), or molasses, to taste

10g torn fresh basil or mint leaves (optional)

fresh mint or basil leaves and a lime wedge, to garnish

Add all of the ingredients (except for the garnish) into a blender and blend until smooth. Taste and add more honey if you like. Pour the drink into a tall glass and garnish with the mint – or basil leaves – and the lime wedge. Serve straight away.

TIP

You can make this slushie with unfrozen watermelon, but you need to add 65–135g ice to the blender. However, with its high water content, watermelon freezes perfectly, so there's really no need for ice: simply flash-freeze cubed watermelon for about 2 hours, then either use them immediately or stash them in a freezer bag for later. You can add a few ice cubes to the blender if you like, but taste the blended mix first, then decide if you'd like a milder flavour.

CITRUS FIZZ

The fizz family of classic cocktails is a tonne of fun to explore. From the Gin Fizz to the New Orleans Fizz, they're well-designed sparkling and foamy drinks filled with flavour. The Citrus Fizz falls nicely into that lineage, and it does have all the style you'd expect – it just skips the booze. It is not a new drink. The recipe is a rendition of one from the mid-twentieth-century, which yields such a great drink that it's worth keeping alive. The Citrus Fizz is a combination of that trifecta of citrus juices: lemon, lime and orange. Add a little grenadine to sweeten up the tart mix, a touch of egg and some sparkling water – and you're done. Wait, an egg? Yes, many classic drinks include an egg. Only use the freshest egg for any drink, though you can also omit it if it doesn't appeal (see Tip). The other trick to a fizz is in the shake. You want to 'dry shake' the base ingredients really well, then add ice, and shake it vigorously a second time. Thanks to the egg, this technique creates that lovely foam, which tops the glass and makes the drink irresistible.

Serves 1

60ml freshly-squeezed
    orange juice
60ml freshly-squeezed
    lemon juice
30ml freshly-squeezed
    lime juice
splash grenadine
1 medium egg (options:
    just the egg white, just
    the yolk – or both)
ice cubes
sparkling water, to fill
1 orange slice, to garnish

Pour the orange, lemon and lime juices, grenadine and egg into a cocktail shaker, then shake the mix for at least 30 seconds. Fill the shaker with ice cubes, and shake for another 30 seconds. Fill a highball glass with ice cubes, strain the cocktail into the glass and slowly pour sparkling water on top to fill. Garnish with the orange slice.

VARIATION

Skip the egg, if you like, and simply have a super-fruity, home-made soft drink.

WATERMELON LEMONADE SPRITZER

When watermelon and lemonade come together, wonderful things happen – and if you top the combination with a little sparkle, a star beverage is born. The Watermelon Lemonade Spritzer is a jug-sized recipe that's perfect for entertaining on the warmest days of the year. Or, simply stock the watermelon lemonade in the fridge and top it with sparkling water any time you like. Watermelon is one of the juiciest fruits you can find. Using a blender and a sieve, it takes little effort to transform it into a liquid. While the juice drains from the pulp, you can whip up a fresh batch of lemonade. Then, when it's time for a drink, pour the beverage into a glass and top it with sparkling or soda water.

Serves 8

1 (2.2kg) watermelon,
    cubed (about 1.2kg)
1 lemon slice and
    1 watermelon wedge
    per serving, to garnish
ice cubes

For the lemonade:
350ml freshly-squeezed
    lemon juice (about 6
    fresh lemons)
240–350ml Simple Syrup
    (see page 13), to taste
475ml sparkling water or
    soda water

Process the watermelon cubes in a blender until smooth. Then press the pulp through a fine-mesh sieve over a bowl to separate the juice from the pulp and seeds (the pulp should be nearly dry when finished). Make the lemonade: combine the lemon juice with 250ml Simple Syrup and 1 litre water. Stir well, add 1 litre watermelon juice, stir again and add more of any desired ingredient. Chill until ready to serve. To serve, pour over ice and top with sparkling or soda water. Garnish with lemon slices and watermelon wedges.

VARIATION

You can also make this spritzer by the glass. Muddle about 6 large cubes of watermelon into a juicy pulp, then strain into a separate glass to remove any seeds. Add about 120ml lemonade and stir well. Fill the glass with ice and top up with some sparkling water.

HOME-MADE GINGER BEER

Ginger beer has a snappy spice that is elevated by carbonation. It's great on its own – and a useful mixer for drinks like the Dark 'n' Blustery (see page 59). The recipe relies on a ginger syrup base (see below) and a few days of fermentation to create a naturally carbonated beverage. While a bit of a chore that requires daily attention, the taste of a home-made ginger beer rivals anything you can buy. With this short fermentation and low sugar content, any alcohol that does develop is negligible.

Serves 6–8

1.8 litres distilled or
   filtered water
150g demerara sugar
150g peeled and minced
   fresh ginger root
120ml freshly-squeezed
   lime or lemon juice
¼ tsp dried champagne
   yeast
ice cubes, to serve
2 or 3 lemon or lime slices
   per serving, to garnish

Bring 1 litre distilled or filtered water to the boil, add the sugar, stir to dissolve. Reduce the heat, add the ginger, simmer for about 5 minutes. Remove the syrup from the heat and cool before straining out the ginger. Stir in the lime or lemon juice, then pour into a 2-litre plastic or glass bottle. Fill the bottle with enough water to leave 5cm of headspace, add the yeast and shake until the yeast is fully dissolved. Add the lid and store in a cool, dark place. Release pressure (next day) by slowly opening the lid. After 2 days, sample a bit of the ginger beer to check for carbonation. Once it's bubbly enough for your taste (this could be up to 4 days, depending on conditions), transfer it to the fridge and enjoy within 2 weeks. (Remember to release the pressure daily.)

VARIATIONS

Demerara sugar adds a deep richness that offsets the ginger spice nicely, though white sugar will work, and soft brown sugar is another option (use an equal amount of dark or light brown sugar). Adjust as required.

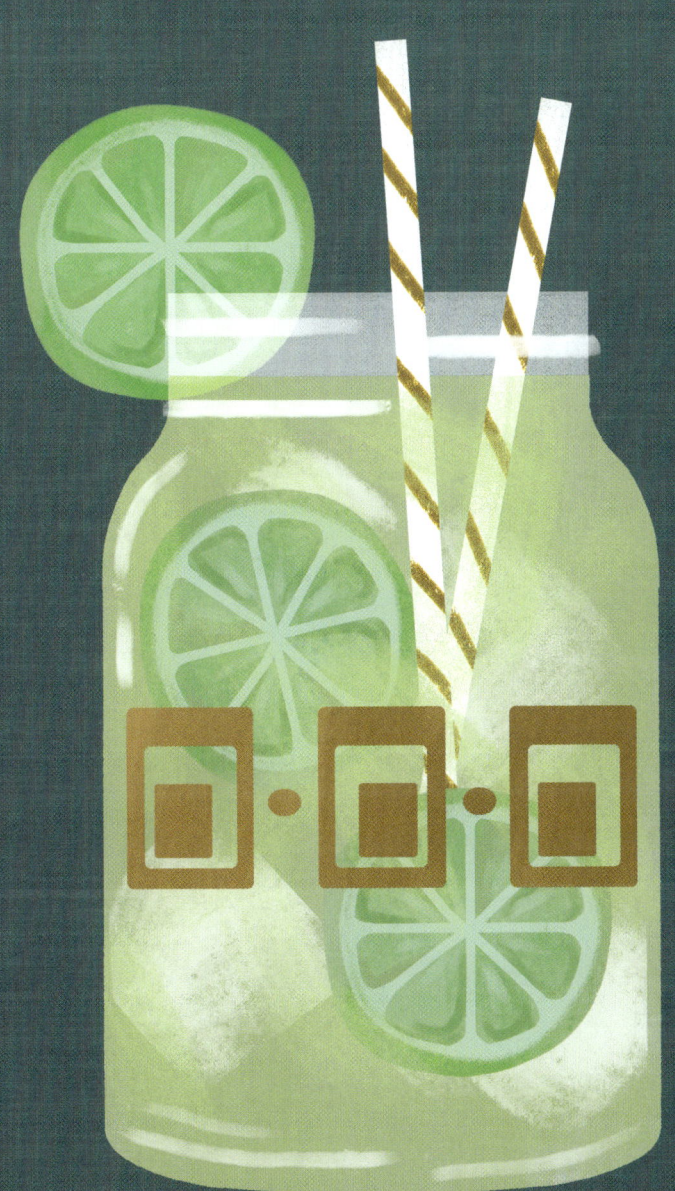

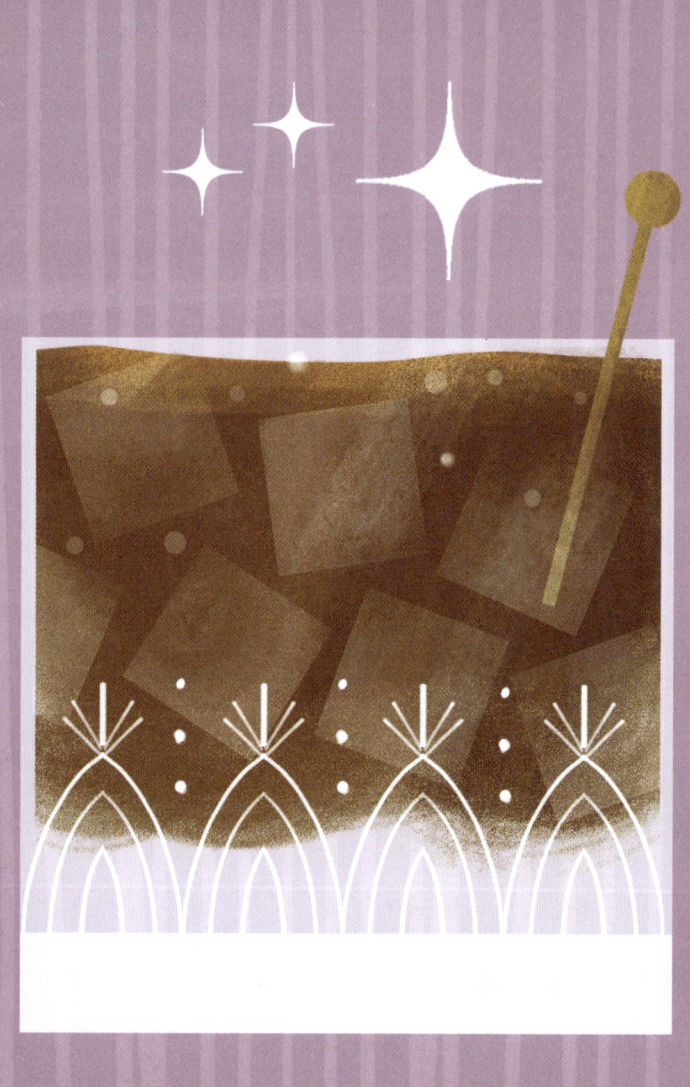

COFFEE 'N' TONIC

While I am generally enamoured with mixed drinks of all kinds, few have truly captured my attention as completely as the combination of really strong coffee and tonic water. At first thought, it seems like some weird anomaly that cannot possibly work. However, once you get a taste of this mix (especially when you need a caffeinated jolt in the middle of the day), the average latte looks like child's play. The key to a good Coffee 'n' Tonic base is strong coffee. Brew the thickest, richest, darkest coffee you can for this drink. If you have an espresso machine, go ahead and pull a shot. A French press or stove-top percolator works, too, and cold-brew coffee is a favourite in this drink. If you just have a regular coffee machine, double or triple the grounds you typically use.

Serves 1

120ml tonic water
ice cubes
60ml strongly brewed
   coffee or espresso,
   chilled

Pour the tonic into a tumbler or highball glass with the ice. Float the coffee over the top, pouring it slowly over the back of a spoon. Stir the drink if you like.

TIP

As with any coffee drink (straight or mixed), it is imperative to start with whole beans that you grind yourself. Each brewing method requires different grind sizes, and you can control this with either an electric or manual grinder.

RASPBERRY-THYME FLORADORA

Named after a Broadway musical from the early 1900s, the Floradora is an utterly delicious, sparkling drink. The original beverage relies on the combination of gin and raspberry liqueur, and it's incredibly easy to make. The key to any Floradora is the sweet taste of raspberries. Rather than a liqueur, we're going with a Raspberry Syrup in this recipe. It's easy to make from fresh or frozen raspberries; just be sure to strain it well to remove all the fruity bits. Thyme is a natural flavour companion and adding it to the muddle is the easiest option, though you can also add a tablespoon of thyme and let it infuse its herbal essence into the syrup. As with many gin-based drinks, you'll want to use a zero-proof gin or non-alcoholic botanical spirit for this one, and I suggest that you play around with the options. A juniper-forward classic gin replica will create an entirely different Floradora than one that is lighter and concentrates on floral flavours. It's really hard to go wrong with either option, and you will find what best suits your taste.

Serves 1

20ml Raspberry Syrup
  (see page 17)
1 tbsp fresh thyme,
  or 1 tsp dried thyme
15ml freshly-squeezed
  lime juice
45ml zero-proof gin
  or non-alcoholic
  botanical spirit
ice cubes
120ml ginger ale (any type)
1 lime wedge, to garnish

Add the Raspberry Syrup, thyme and lime juice to a highball glass, and muddle well. Pour in the non-alcoholic botanical spirit, fill the glass with ice, then top with the ginger ale. Stir the drink well. Garnish with the lime wedge.

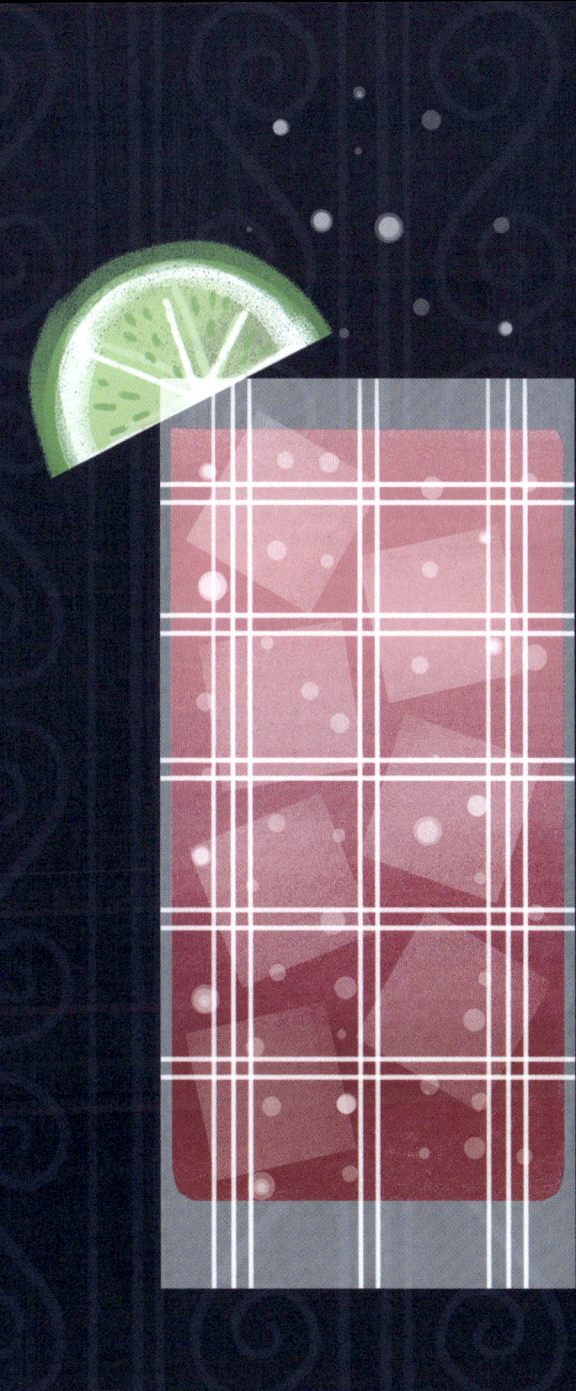

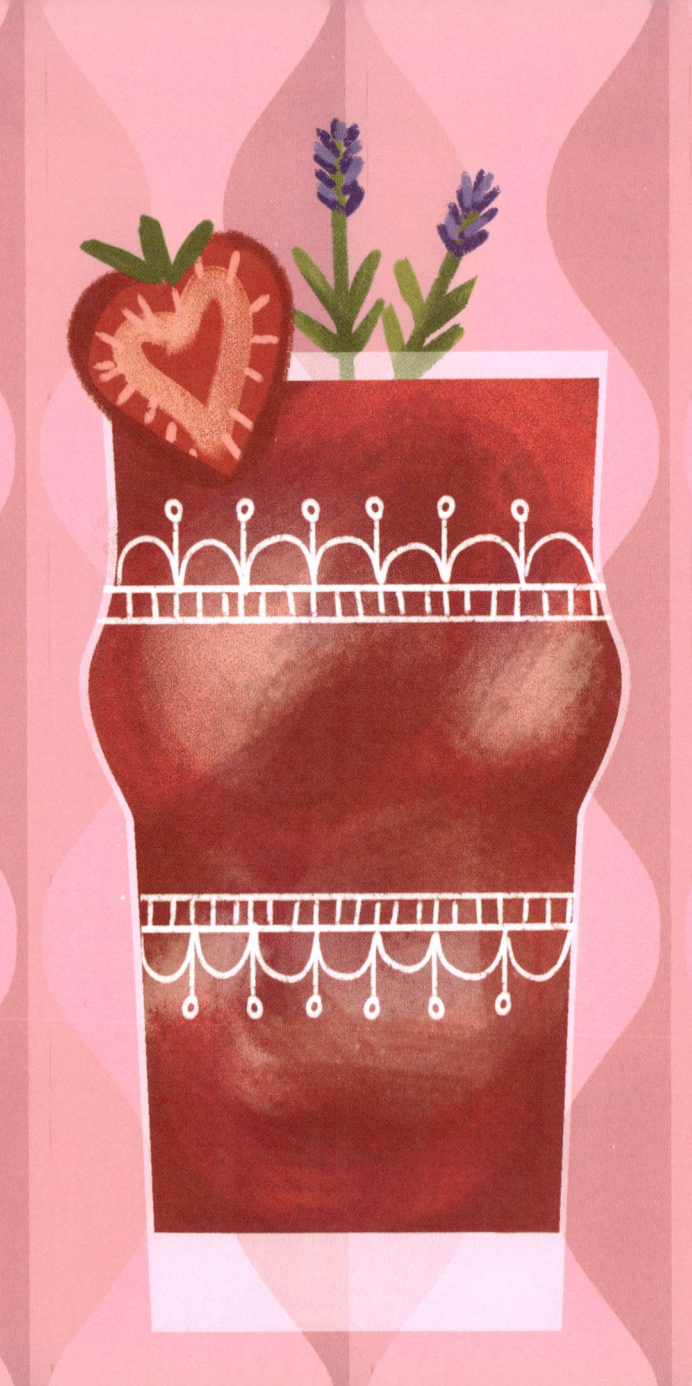

STRAWBERRY–HIBISCUS AGUA FRESCA

Refreshing and the perfect large-batch beverage for a hot day, agua fresca is not to be overlooked. The name is Spanish for 'fresh water', and that translation describes it wonderfully – it is neither juice nor flavoured water, it is the best of both! Requiring nothing more than fruit, water and sugar, the possibilities of this drink are nearly endless. What fruit do you have in the fridge, or what looks fabulous at the market right now? Melons are a popular option, as are berries, peaches and pineapple, though don't stop there! Some of the more classic agua fresca flavours in Mexico are as diverse and exciting as tamarind, hibiscus and horchata. There are no rules in agua fresca!

Serves 6

20g dried hibiscus
  flowers
280g sliced strawberries
  or other fresh fruit
  (see headnote)
60ml Lavender-honey
  Syrup (see page 14),
  Rosemary Syrup
  (see page 15) or agave
  nectar, or to taste
30ml fresh lime juice,
  or to taste
1 fresh strawberry, and
  1 lavender or rosemary
  sprig per serving,
  to garnish
ice cubes

Bring 1.5 litres water to the boil, then remove from the heat and add the hibiscus flowers. Cover and steep until cool, then strain out the hibiscus. Add the hibiscus tea, strawberries, syrup and lime juice to a blender, and purée until smooth. Taste, and add more syrup or citrus as needed, blending again. Run it through a fine-mesh sieve to remove any fruit pulp. Refrigerate until chilled, and serve over ice (it keeps well for about a week). Garnish, using strawberries and lavender or rosemary sprigs, as you prefer.

VARIATIONS

Try various simple syrups (see pages 12–13). Mint is rather versatile for most fruits, but also try a jalapeño syrup in a pineapple agua fresca – it's a fabulous flavour pairing!

SAGE SOUR

The Sour is a classic cocktail formula featuring a spirit (whisky, rum, gin or tequila), sweetener and citrus fruit. When you find the perfect balance of those three elements, a beautiful drink is yours to enjoy. Try the Sage Sour with a zero-proof whisky or dark rum. If you don't have either of those, replace them with an extra pour of apple juice, which is a fantastic pairing for the Sage Syrup and lemon juice. It's a great dinner beverage in the autumn, and goes really well with a holiday feast. Choose a high-quality apple juice (or make it yourself, see page 31), or go with apple cider for this one.

Serves 1

ice cubes
60ml zero-proof
  whisky or dark rum
  (see headnote)
30ml apple juice
30ml Sage Syrup
  (see page 17)
15ml freshly-squeezed
  lemon juice
1 lemon twist or sage
  leaf, to garnish

Into a cocktail shaker filled with the ice, pour the ingredients. Shake vigorously, then strain into a chilled cocktail or coupe glass. Garnish with the lemon twist or sage leaf.

SUMMER CUP MOCKTAIL

The Wimbledon tennis tournament is synonymous with a drink called a Pimm's Cup. It mixes a liqueur – called Pimm's No. 1 – with lemonade, cucumber, berries and a bit of mint or orange here and there. This simultaneously refreshing and original beverage has been a summer-time favourite since the 1800s! For this Summer Cup Mocktail of the free-spirited world, you'll need to stock up on fruits: oranges, lemons, limes, strawberries and a cucumber are essential (other berries work, too), and some fresh mint may also please you. Primarily, you need to perfect your home-made lemonade skills – that is non-negotiable. Another surprising cameo is made by balsamic vinegar. Somehow, it really works, and finishes it all off with a surprising flourish.

Serves 6

1 sprig mint, leaves only
1 orange, for 6 slices of about 3–5mm thick
6 strawberries, hulled and sliced lengthways
½ medium cucumber, sliced
1 lemon, sliced
1 litre home-made lemonade (see page 85)
1 tbsp balsamic vinegar
ice cubes
any leftover (or extra) fruit or mint, to garnish

In a jug, add the fruits, lemonade and balsamic vinegar. Stir well and refrigerate for 3–4 hours to let the flavours meld. To serve, pour into ice-filled glasses and add extra fruit slices or mint as a garnish. The real beauty of this drink is that there's no mixing. Stirring in the balsamic is key – but, other than that, the fruits naturally infuse the drink. It gets better the longer the flavours meld, which is why I created this as a jug drink – think sangria with a British twist.

VARIATIONS

For a bit of sparkle, top each glass with a splash of soda water or ginger ale. Rather than just strawberries, use a combination of summer berries. Freeze some as an alternative to ice.

CUCUMBER–MINT COOLER

If it hasn't already, the combination of cucumber and mint is sure to capture your taste buds and become a lifelong favourite. In this cooler, the dynamic duo is accented by home-made lemonade (see page 85) and the non-alcoholic gin or booze-free botanical spirit of your choice. When it comes to choosing the zero-proof gin or a non-alcoholic, botanical spirit for this drink, you'll likely find that the softer, the better. This mocktail is stellar with 'spirits' that are focused on floral and citrus flavours, rather than the spiced replicas of a classic London dry gin. Better yet, if you come across a bottle that promotes cucumber (similar to Hendrick's), pour that – you won't regret it!

Serves 1

3 slices cucumber, about 3mm thick
2 slices green apple (optional)
6 fresh mint leaves
45ml zero-proof gin or non-alcoholic botanical spirit
ice cubes
120–150ml home-made lemonade (see page 85)
1 lemon, apple or cucumber slice, and 1 mint sprig, to garnish

In a highball glass, muddle the cucumber, apple and mint, then add the spirit. Fill the glass with the ice, top with lemonade and stir well. Garnish with lemon, apple or cucumber slices, and finish with a mint sprig.

VARIATIONS

Top this one with sparkling lemon soda or tonic water – for a little sparkle.

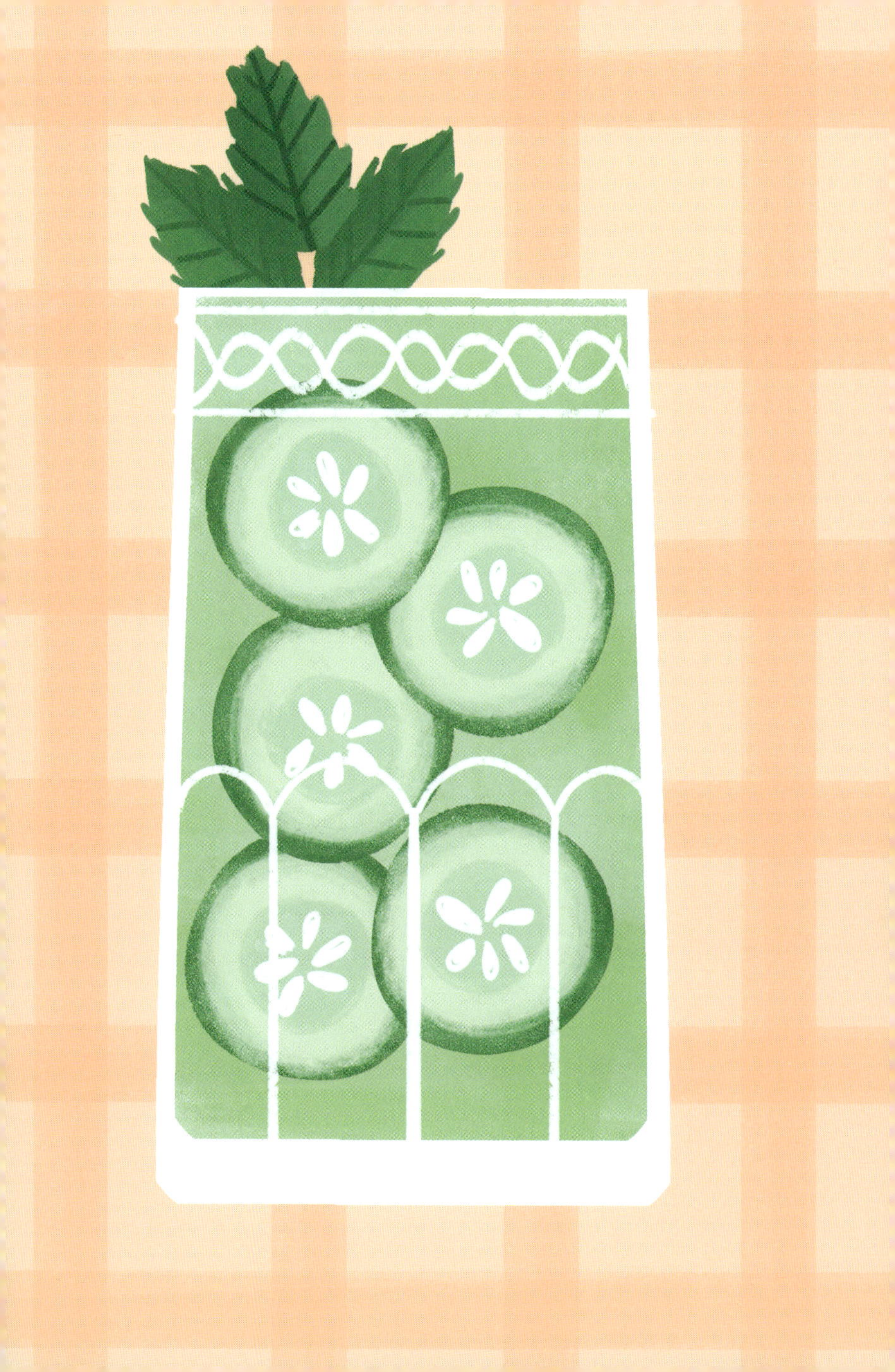

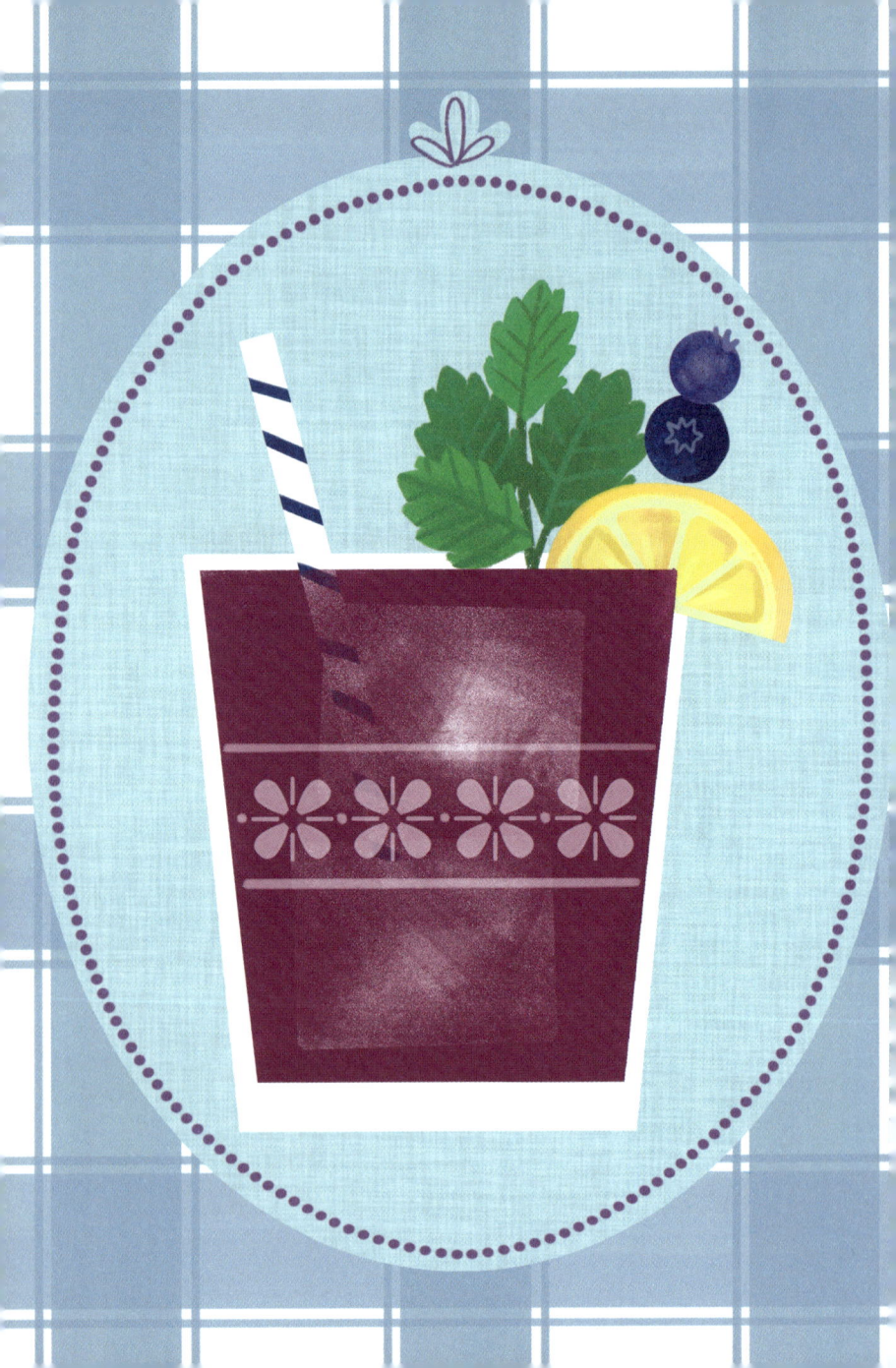

BLUEBERRY-MINT SMASH

Smash cocktails are exactly what they sound like: you smash ingredients with a muddler. They're fun and fruity, and make great sippers for a casual afternoon drink. Taking a tip from the whisky smash, this recipe combines fresh blueberries, mint and lemon. The trio takes the edge off the often-spicy zero-proof whisky, and creates a pleasant mocktail. The home-made almond syrup really brings everything together, and it's incredibly easy to make (see Tip). If you have blueberry preserves, about two teaspoons makes a good substitute for fresh blueberries. This drink is also excellent when topped with a bit of soda water or tonic, if you're looking for something a bit taller and more refreshing.

Serves 1

2 lemon wedges
6–8 fresh mint leaves
8–10 fresh blueberries
   or 2 tsp blueberry
   preserve (see headnote)
½ tbsp almond syrup
   (see Tip)
ice cubes
60ml zero-proof whisky
soda or tonic water, to top
   (optional, see headnote)
1 fresh mint sprig,
   1 lemon slice and
   3–5 blueberries,
   to garnish

In an old-fashioned glass, muddle the lemon, mint and blueberries with the almond syrup. Fill the glass with the ice, add the zero-proof whisky and stir well. Garnish with the mint, lemon and blueberries.

TIP

To create an almond syrup, simply add two teaspoons of almond extract to the regular Simple Syrup recipe (see page 13).

SPICE 'N' TONIC

Tonic water is an ideal base for a bit of spice, and it works fabulously with apple cider to create a beautiful and refreshing autumn drink. The spiciness of zero-proof whisky is a great base for this recipe. However, there are several zero-proof gins or non-alcoholic botanical spirits that promote a spice-forward flavour profile (they'll often have the word 'spice' in their name), and these are an equally good option for this tonic. There's really no mixing required, but you'll want to let this rest for a minute or two before consuming its delights. As it sits, the cinnamon, cloves, star anise and orange infuse the drink with their inviting array of flavours, and this makes the drink that much better.

Serves 1

ice cubes
60ml zero-proof whisky,
   gin or botanical spirit
30ml apple cider
120ml tonic water
1 cinnamon stick
3 cloves
1 star anise
1 orange slice

Into a highball glass filled with the ice, pour the spirit and cider, and stir well. Top with the tonic water, then drop the cinnamon stick, cloves, star anise and orange slice into the glass to add their unique flavour influences to the drink.

VARIATION

For a hint of sweetness and a bit more spice, add 15ml spiced brown sugar syrup (see Warming Winter Cup recipe, page 141).

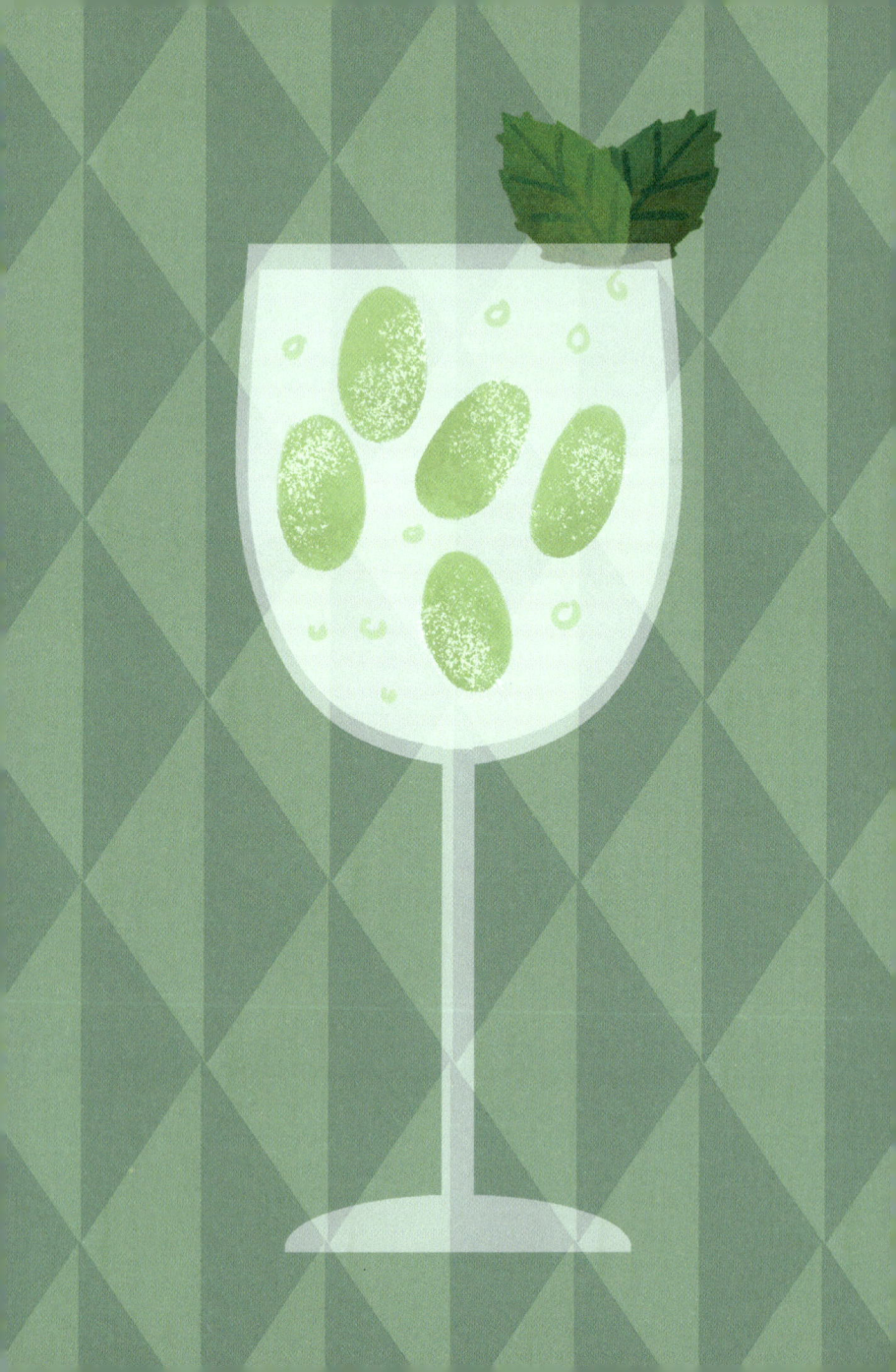

WHITE GRAPE SUNDOWNER

The Sundowner is one of my favourite mocktails of all time. I've made it regularly for a couple of decades, and it's even more interesting today thanks to the non-alcoholic botanical spirit options. I'd strongly recommend those with a floral or citrus dominance, as they'll play nicely with the grape juice and sparkling water or wine. White grape juice is key to a Sundowner. While not one of the most prevalent juices, you should find it at a decent supermarket. The taste is light, refreshing and perfectly sweet – close to a white wine. Try flavoured sparkling water or use the Sundowner to explore non-alcoholic sparkling wines. The frozen grapes are the final puzzle piece to this drink; green or red will work, though I prefer green. They play the role of ice cubes, keeping your drink chilled, and they look fabulous floating in the glass.

Serves 1

5–6 frozen grapes
45ml zero-proof gin or non-alcoholic botanical spirit
90ml white grape juice
90ml flavoured sparkling water or non-alcoholic sparkling wine
2–3 fresh mint leaves, to garnish

Place the frozen grapes in a white wine glass or champagne flute. Add the spirit and juice, and top with sparkling water or non-alcoholic wine. Add the fresh mint leaves as a garnish.

CINDERELLA

A trio of fruit juices, a splash of grenadine and a ginger ale or beer creates the timeless mocktail known as the Cinderella. As lovely as its name, this concoction makes you want to pop on your glass slippers and meet up with your Prince (or Princess) Charming. The ginger aspect is key to this simple mocktail. For a lightly sweetened, sparkling touch, seek out a good-quality ginger ale. When you're in the mood for something a bit bolder, ginger beer is the way to go (see page 86 for a home-made recipe). If neither is at your disposal, sparkling or soda water will do. Fresh lemon and orange juices are essential. Unless you have an electric juicer, creating fresh pineapple juice is not so simple. However, if you have a blender and a sieve (for removing the pineapple pulp), it is possible. Give it a go! You can save any leftovers for other pineapple drinks, such as the Virgin Piña Colada (see page 36).

Serves 1

ice cubes
30ml freshly-squeezed
  lemon juice
30ml freshly-squeezed
  orange juice
30ml fresh or bottled
  pineapple juice (see
  headnote)
15ml grenadine
60ml ginger ale, ginger
  beer, soda water or
  sparkling water
  (see headnote)
1 pineapple wedge and
  1 orange slice, to garnish

Into a highball glass filled with the ice, pour the lemon, orange and pineapple juices, plus the grenadine. Stir well, then top with the ginger ale or ginger beer. Garnish with the pineapple wedge and orange slice.

VARIATIONS

Add a shot (45ml) of a floral or fruity, non-alcoholic botanical spirit.

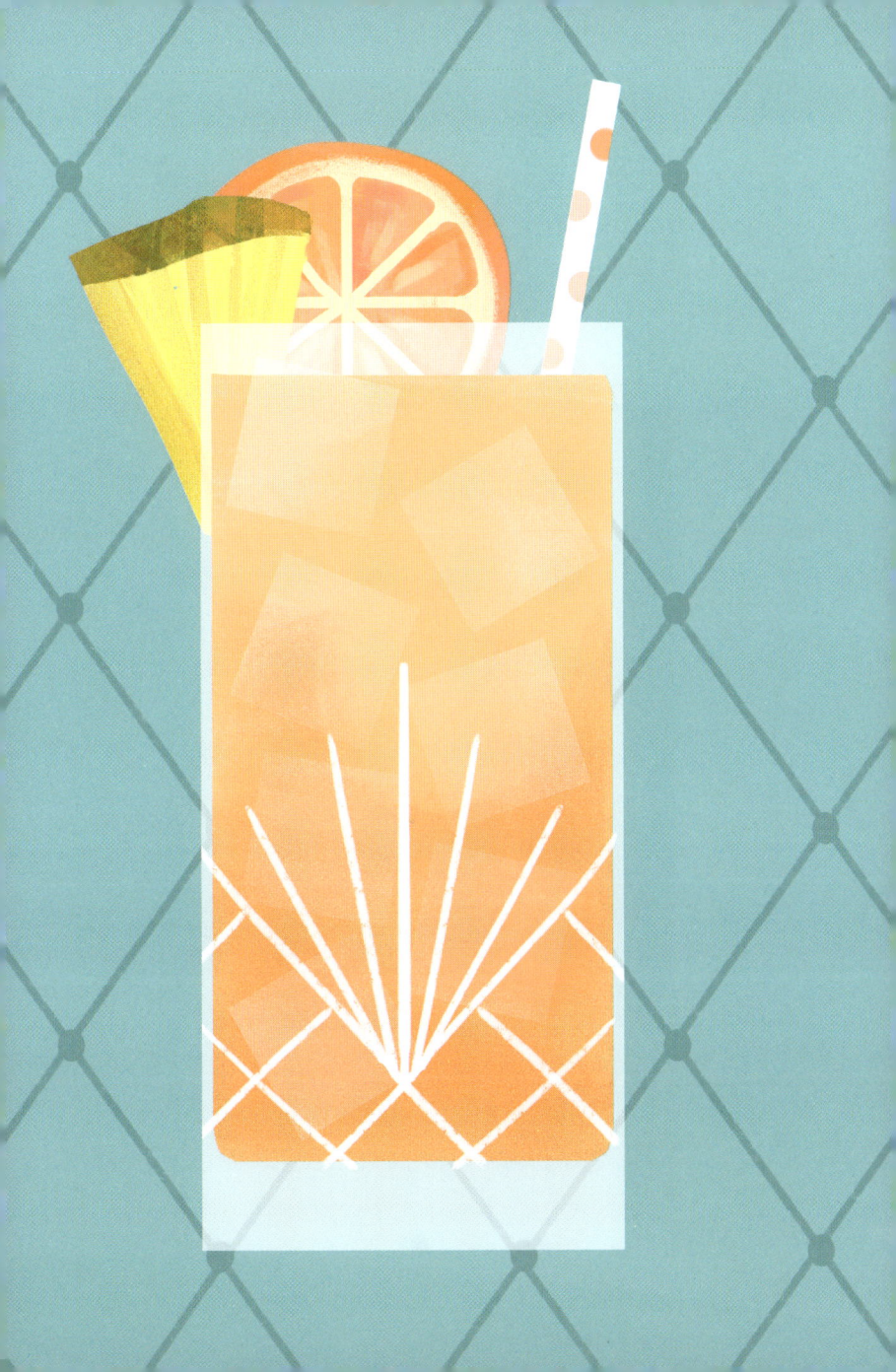

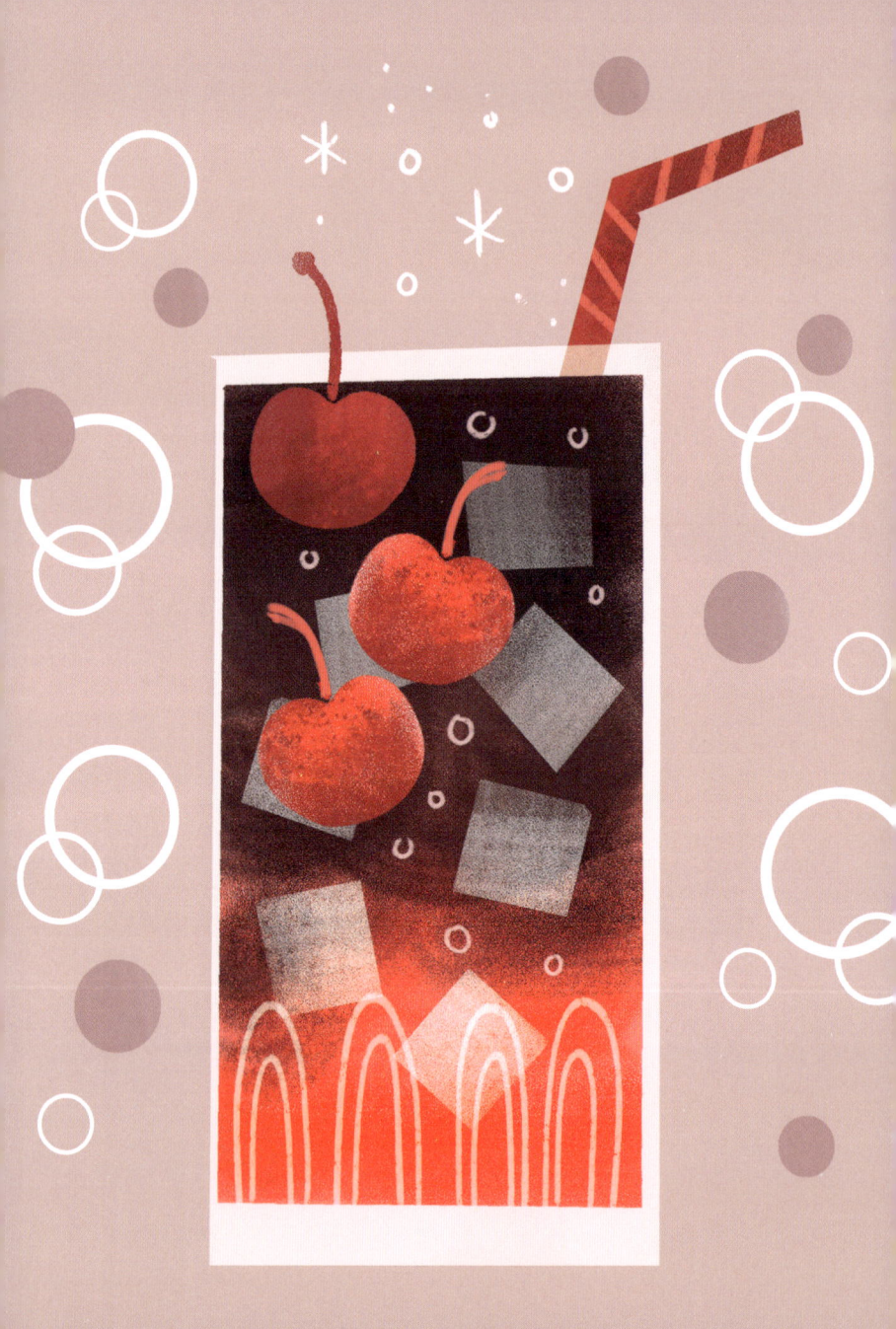

ROY ROGERS

If you love the Shirley Temple (see page 78), this beverage is essentially the same thing, but with a cola twist. It's crazily easy to make, which is why it's long been a favourite among the non-drinking crowd. This classic, old-school mocktail is named after the 'King of the Cowboys' and ultimate 'good guy', Roy Rogers. Traditionally, the Roy Rogers is made with Coca-Cola (or Pepsi, at bars that prefer to serve that brand). However, I encourage you to get a better taste of this drink with the boutique soft drink brands that use the real kola nut (Fever-Tree is one of my long-standing favourites, but there are others). These beverages are significantly less sweet than what the 'big guys' offer, and they offer a really nice level of spice in their flavour balance. Therefore, the grenadine plays much better against these less sweetened products. If you do pour a sweeter cola, though – cut the grenadine in half.

Serves 1

ice cubes
30ml grenadine
180ml cola (see headnote)
3 fresh or maraschino
   cherries, to garnish

Fill a highball glass with the ice and pour in the grenadine. Top with the cola, then garnish your drink with the cherries.

VARIATIONS

Add a shot (45ml) of a non-alcoholic whisky or rum. The sweetness of the other ingredients will create a perfectly balanced drink against the zero-proof spirit's spiciness.

WHIPPED LEMONADE

Whipped Lemonade, which started as a social media trend, is now a huge hit and viral sensation. In reality, this drink is little more than a lemon milkshake, but it is delicious, so get ready and pull out your blender for this one! There are several ways to make Whipped Lemonade, and none of them will disappoint. Using regular cream is a popular option, but we're taking the vegan route in this recipe and using coconut, because cream of coconut makes a wonderful base for the tart taste of fresh lemon juice. (On the lemon front, bottled lemon juice simply can't compete with freshly squeezed juice.)

Serves 2

600g crushed ice
250ml freshly-squeezed
   lemon juice
225g cream of coconut
1 lemon wedge and
   1 fresh mint sprig
   per glass (optional),
   to garnish

Place the ice in a blender, then add the lemon juice and cream of coconut. Blend until smooth, then pour into a frosty highball glass and add the lemon wedge and mint sprig to garnish.

VARIATIONS

Substitute the cream of coconut with double cream. Even whole milk or coconut milk will work, though you'll want to add less ice at first, then add more as needed to get the desired consistency. Add some fruits to the mix – strawberries and pineapple are amazing additions to a home-made Whipped Lemonade!

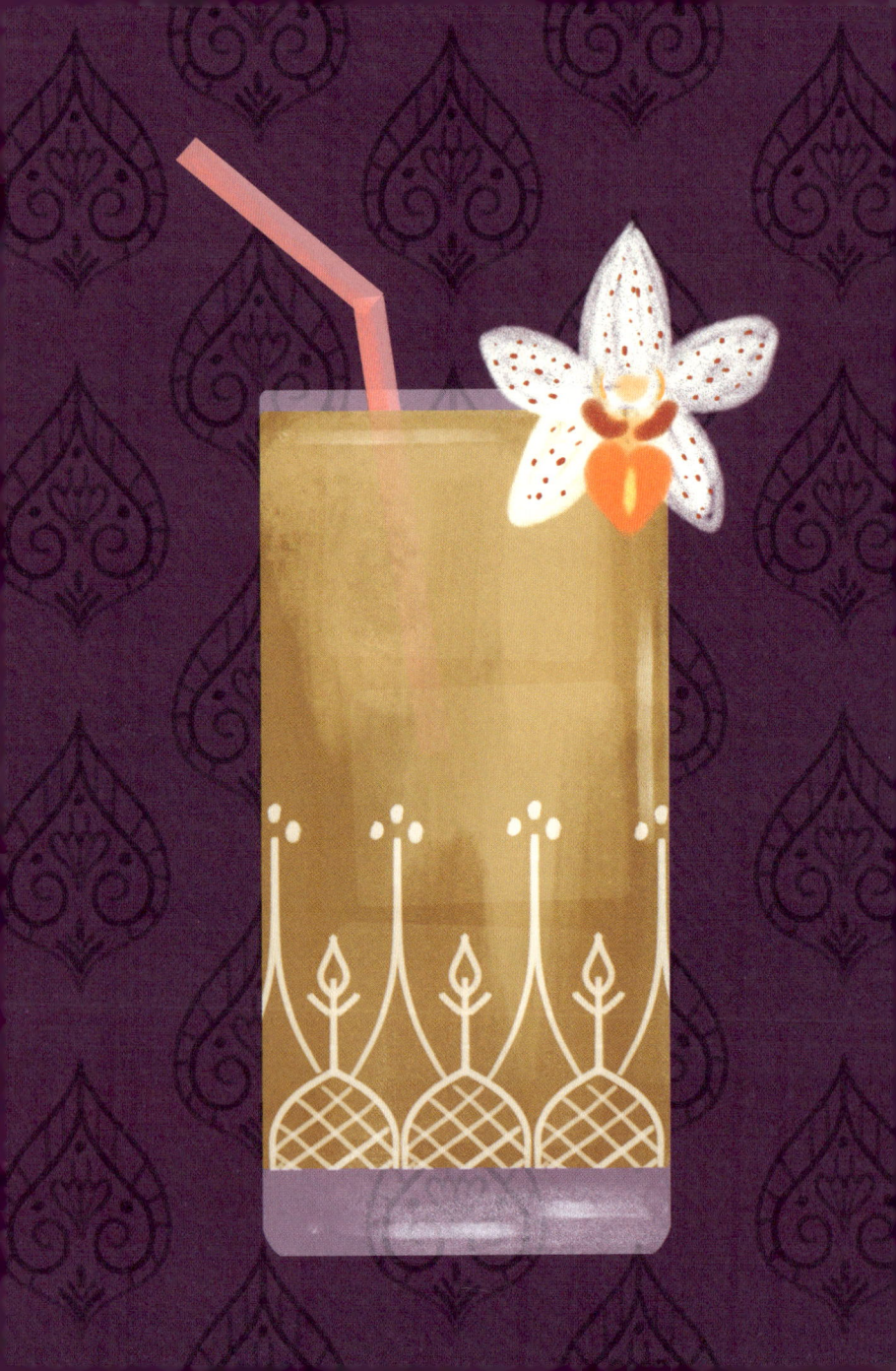

THAI ICED TEA

Let's take a look at a brilliant tea drink that would put any Long Island Iced Tea to shame. Thai Iced Tea is simply delicious, and making it from scratch is neither difficult nor a waste of time. All you need is a well-stocked spice cupboard and your favourite black tea. Essentially, this drink is spiced black tea, which is then chilled, poured over ice and topped with milk. Considering the spices, it's best made as a double serving, though you can store the brewed, spiced tea in a well-sealed glass jar – in the fridge – for a day or two.

Serves 2

2 tbsp black tea leaves
1 star anise
2 cardamom pods
1 cinnamon stick
¼ tsp pure almond
  extract
1 tbsp granulated
  sugar
15ml sweetened
  condensed milk
ice cubes
15ml full-fat coconut
  or whole milk

Bring 250ml water to the boil, then add the tea leaves, star anise, cardamom, cinnamon and almond extract. Stir, then steep for 5 minutes. Strain out the tea and the spices. Stir in the sugar and sweetened condensed milk until dissolved, and let the mix cool for a few minutes. Pour the tea into ice-filled glasses, then slowly pour the coconut or whole milk over the top.

VARIATIONS

Vanilla extract will work in this recipe if you don't have any almond extract available. You can top this drink with extra sweetened condensed milk if you have some. For a vegan option, switch from sweetened condensed milk to cream of coconut.

SWEET PEPPER SPRITZER

Allow me to introduce you to the wonders of a juiced pepper. Too often, we think these sweet peppers should be reserved for food, but with the help of your muddler, magic happens! I really didn't believe it myself until I tried it and developed a straight-from-the-garden mocktail. Give it a shot, and you might be surprised! Red peppers are the ideal option for this drink, but if you have green or orange peppers, those will work. These peppers produce a surprising amount of juice under the power of a muddler, and pair wonderfully with fresh herbs. If you have both herbs available, the combo of muddled basil and a thyme garnish will nicely enhance this drink, though either will work as substitutes for one another.

Serves 2

1 medium red, green or
  orange pepper, sliced
  (see headnote)
5 fresh basil leaves
  or thyme sprig
  (see headnote)
3 tbsp freshly-squeezed
  lemon juice
1 tbsp agave nectar
ice cubes
150ml ginger ale, or
  to taste
1 lemon slice and 1 fresh
  basil or thyme sprig per
  glass, to garnish

In an old-fashioned glass or highball glass, muddle the pepper, basil, lemon juice and agave nectar thoroughly (it should take just a minute or two) to release all of the pepper's juices and the basil's essence. Fill the glass with the ice, top with ginger ale – then garnish with the lemon slices and fresh basil or thyme.

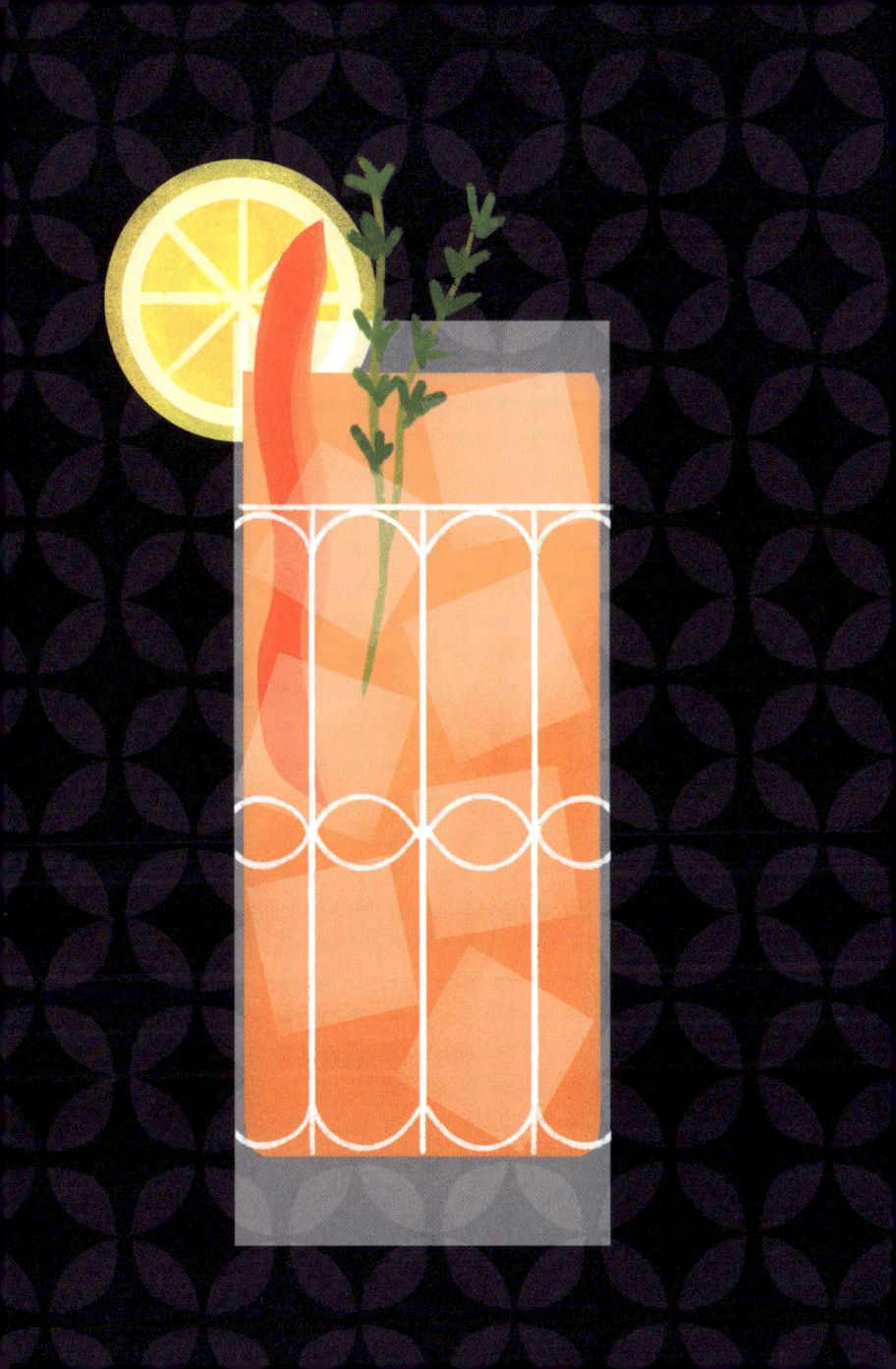

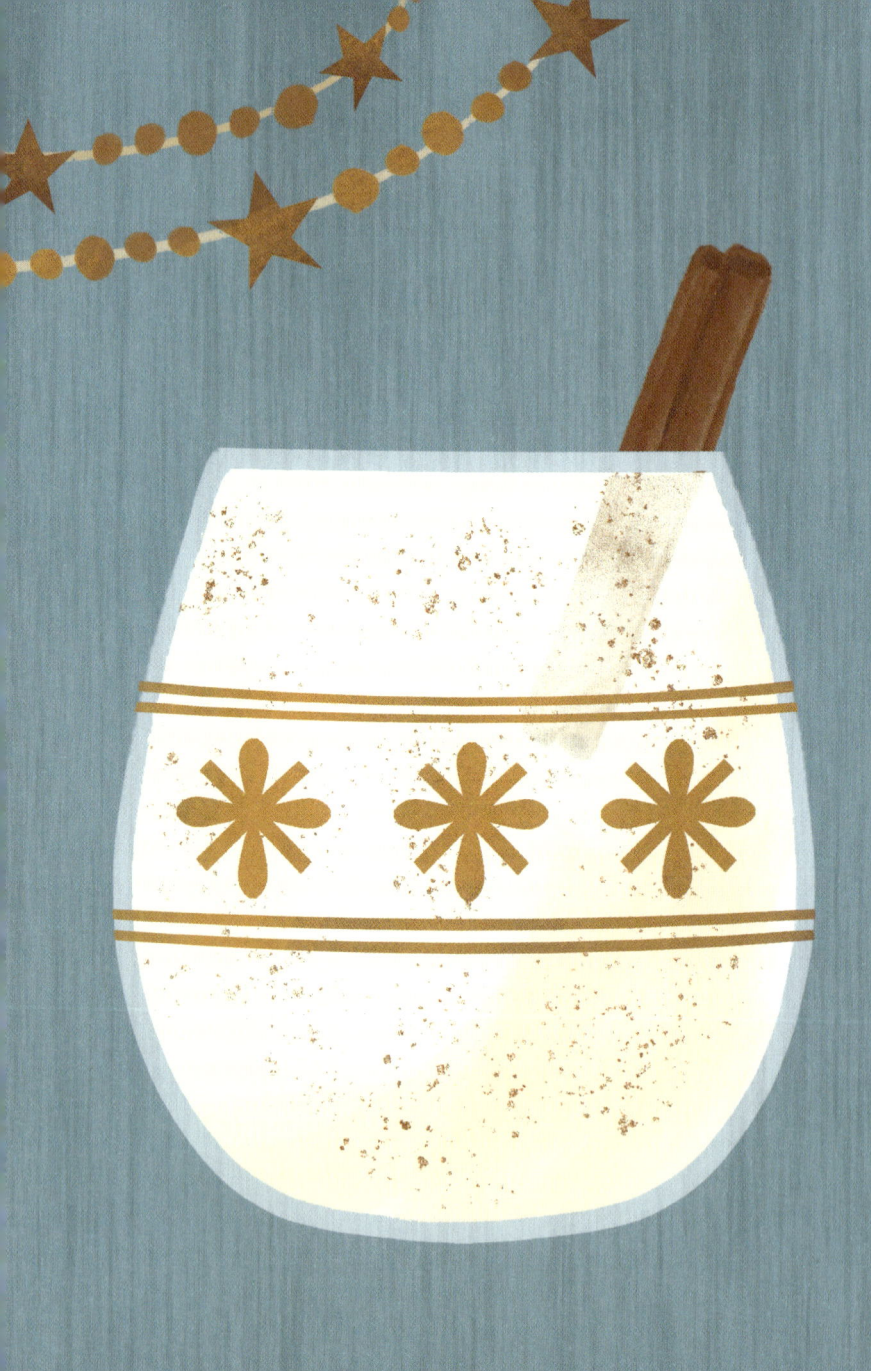

VEGAN EGGNOG

When the holidays roll around and you want a classic beverage, few drinks satisfy like eggnog. While eggs really do put the 'egg' in the nog, there is a vegan option: tofu. Along with almond milk, tofu creates a festive drink that is just as satisfying and lusciously thick as genuine eggnog. Adding a non-alcoholic rum or whisky gives the drink depth, as the spirit's inherent flavours and botanicals play wonderfully off the spices. The key to any great eggnog (vegan or not) is to let it rest. Give it at least an hour before you consume it. It tastes even better if you have the patience to make it 24 hours in advance of supping, as this allows the flavours to develop and marry over a whole day.

Serves 8

680g silken tofu, crumbled
475ml almond milk
70g golden sugar,
  or to taste
¼ tsp sea salt
4 tsp pure vanilla extract
½ tsp grated nutmeg
½ tsp ground cinnamon
250ml non-alcoholic rum
  or whisky (optional)
135–165g ice cubes,
  or as needed
1 cinnamon stick and pinch
  of grated nutmeg per
  glass, to garnish

Purée the tofu, almond milk, sugar and salt in a blender until smooth. Whisk in the vanilla, nutmeg, cinnamon and the non-alcoholic rum or whiskey, if using. Cover and refrigerate for 1–24 hours. When ready to serve, blend again with the ice cubes. Serve, garnishing with the cinnamon sticks and a dusting of nutmeg.

CARROT-GINGER REVITALIZER

Carrot juice is a rather surprising cocktail ingredient that is filled with nutritious benefits. The carrot pairs well with ginger and lemon, creating a most delightful drink. In order to offset the savoury flavour, a bit of Honey Syrup adds a touch of sweetness, while soda water gives it sparkle and creates an ultra-refreshing drink. To introduce a slight ginger-like bite, I add a pinch of ground turmeric to the drink.

Serves 1

ice cubes
120ml carrot juice
½ tsp grated ginger
¼ tsp ground
    turmeric (optional)
2 tsp Honey Syrup
    (see page 14)
1 tbsp freshly-squeezed
    lemon juice
120ml soda water or
    sparkling water
1 lemon slice, to garnish

In a cocktail shaker filled with ice, combine the carrot juice, ginger, turmeric, syrup and lemon juice. Shake well, then strain into a chilled glass over fresh ice. Top with soda water, and garnish with the lemon slice.

VARIATIONS

Add 60ml zero-proof rum. Alternatively, using beetroot juice (about 60ml of it) adds a fun twist.

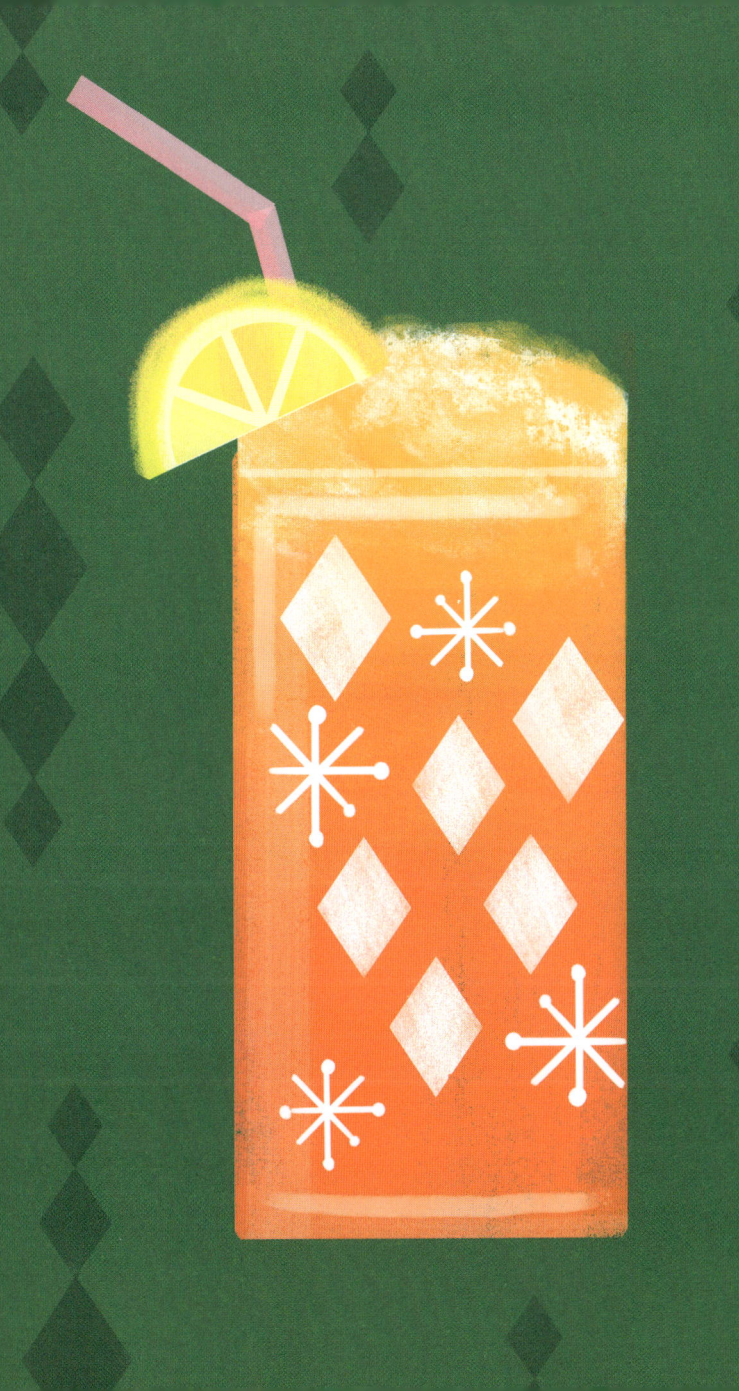

KEY LIME PIE LIMEADE

The Key Lime Pie, a vodka-based Martini, is so deliciously tantalizing that it's far too easy to drink one too many. In the spirit of that drink, this home-made limeade is a good alternative. Every element that makes the cocktail and pie fantastic is included, it's just slightly more refreshing and far less indulgent (both in sugar and alcohol!). The real key to this drink is to make a sweetener-free lime cordial from scratch. Key limes are not as plentiful or juicy as regular limes, but if you have the opportunity to use them, go for it. Once the cordial is made, a bit of pineapple juice, Vanilla-orange Syrup – and a hint of soda water sparkle – transform this drink into a refreshing summer beverage worthy of any barbecue.

Serves 1

1 lime wedge, for the rim
   and to garnish
crushed digestive biscuits,
   for the rim (optional)
ice cubes
60ml Vanilla-orange
   Syrup (see page 16)
30ml home-made Lime
   Cordial (see right)
30ml pineapple juice
45ml non-alcoholic
   botanical spirit (optional)
30ml club sparkling or
   soda water, or to taste

Wipe the rim of an old-fashioned glass with a lime wedge, and roll it in a small dish of finely crushed digestive biscuits. Into a cocktail shaker filled with ice, pour the syrup, Lime Cordial, pineapple juice and non-alcoholic botanical spirit. Shake well, then strain into the prepared glass and add a splash of soda water. Garnish with the lime wedge.

Lime Cordial (makes 2 cups)
¾ tsp citric acid
½ tsp tartaric acid (optional)
150g white granulated sugar
grated zest and freshly-squeezed juice of
   3 limes or key limes (about 150ml juice)

Bring 350ml water to the boil, then stir in the citric acid, tartaric acid and sugar until dissolved. Remove from the heat, and add the lime zest and juice. Cover, let steep until cool. Thanks to its citric acid, lime cordial stores very well. Stored in an airtight container, in the fridge, it can last up to 4 months.

TEA NON-TINI

Brew a cup of tea, chill it, mix it and serve it up with a lemon garnish, and you have a simple variation on a Tea Tini. For this recipe, you can choose any tea or herb you have available. Jasmine tea makes a lovely drink, as does any other green tea. Hibiscus tea creates a nice floral option, while herbal teas work just as well. When you switch from the Tea Tini's usual vodka to a non-alcoholic botanical spirit, it's an equally pleasing mocktail. I do like a sugar rim on this one because it adds the ideal amount of sweetness and makes the drink feel a bit fancier.

Serves 1

1 lemon slice or twist, for
    the rim and to garnish
granulated sugar, for
    the rim
ice cubes
45ml zero-proof gin
    or non-alcoholic
    botanical spirit
60ml chilled, brewed
    tea (see headnote)
7.5ml freshly-squeezed
    lemon juice
1 tsp Simple or Honey
    Syrup (see pages
    13 and 14)

Rim a cocktail glass with sugar by wetting the rim with the lemon slice, then rolling it in a shallow dish of sugar. Into a cocktail shaker filled with the ice, pour the spirit, tea, lemon juice and syrup. Shake well, strain into the prepared glass and garnish with the lemon slice or twist.

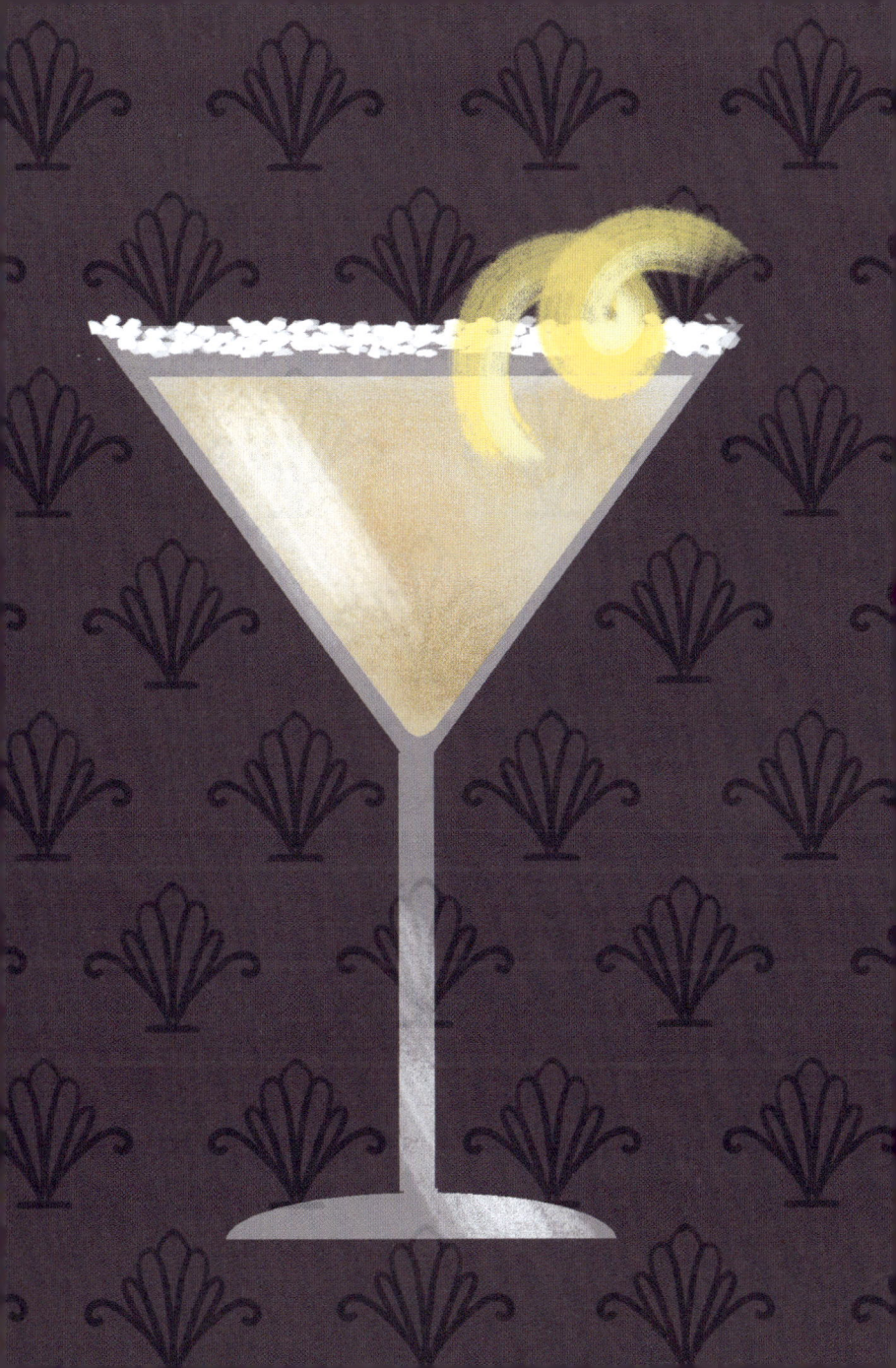

HOT BUTTERED APPLE CIDER

When winter rolls around, few drinks are as comforting as whisky or a hot buttered rum. That said, apple cider also does the trick. This drink requires a spiced buttered batter, using nothing more than sugar, butter, a hint of sweetener and a variety of warming spices. Make the batter and let it rest in the fridge for at least an hour, although the flavours meld far better after 24 hours. If you want to store it for longer than that, put your seasoned butter 'log' in the freezer, then let it thaw before using it.

Serves 1

60ml apple cider
30ml Buttered Batter,
   or to taste (see right)
90–120ml hot (not boiling)
   water, or to taste
1 cinnamon stick,
   to garnish

When ready to build the drink, place a dollop of the Buttered Batter into a mug, then add the apple cider and top with hot water. Garnish with the cinnamon stick.

Buttered Batter (serves 12)
150g brown sugar
115g unsalted butter, at room
   temperature
60g agave nectar
½ tsp ground cinnamon
¼ tsp ground allspice
¼ tsp ground cloves
¼ tsp ground nutmeg
pinch sea salt

Combine all of the ingredients in a small bowl, stirring until well incorporated. Form the batter into a log and encase with clingfilm; refrigerate for 1–24 hours, or freeze for up to 3 months.

VARIATIONS

Add a shot of zero-proof rum or whisky along with the batter before building the drink. For extra flavour, brew a black tea and use that instead of water.

AUTUMNAL TEMPTATIONS

You know that day when it feels like summer's over and winter's going to bring its blustery nastiness in at any moment, but then you get a glimpse of warm sunshine that makes you want to forget every obligation? Yeah, it was exactly like that when I created this drink, and that's why it's called Autumnal 'Temptations'. Apricot nectar, along with a hint of grapefruit juice and just a dash of agave nectar for sweetness, is a beautiful thing. However, the 'temptation' in this drink really comes with the sparkle. While rare, lavender water truly sets this mocktail off (you can make your own by mixing soda water with a Lavender-honey Syrup – see page 14). Yet, plain soda water will do just as well. With either option, this sparkler will have you wanting to jet right out of the office to soak up those last bits of afternoon sun!

Serves 1

ice cubes
90ml apricot nectar
½ tbsp agave nectar
60ml grapefruit juice
60–90ml lavender fizzy
  water, soda water or
  sparkling water

Into a highball glass filled with the ice, pour the apricot and agave nectars, plus the grapefruit juice. Stir well, then top up with soda (or sparkling) water.

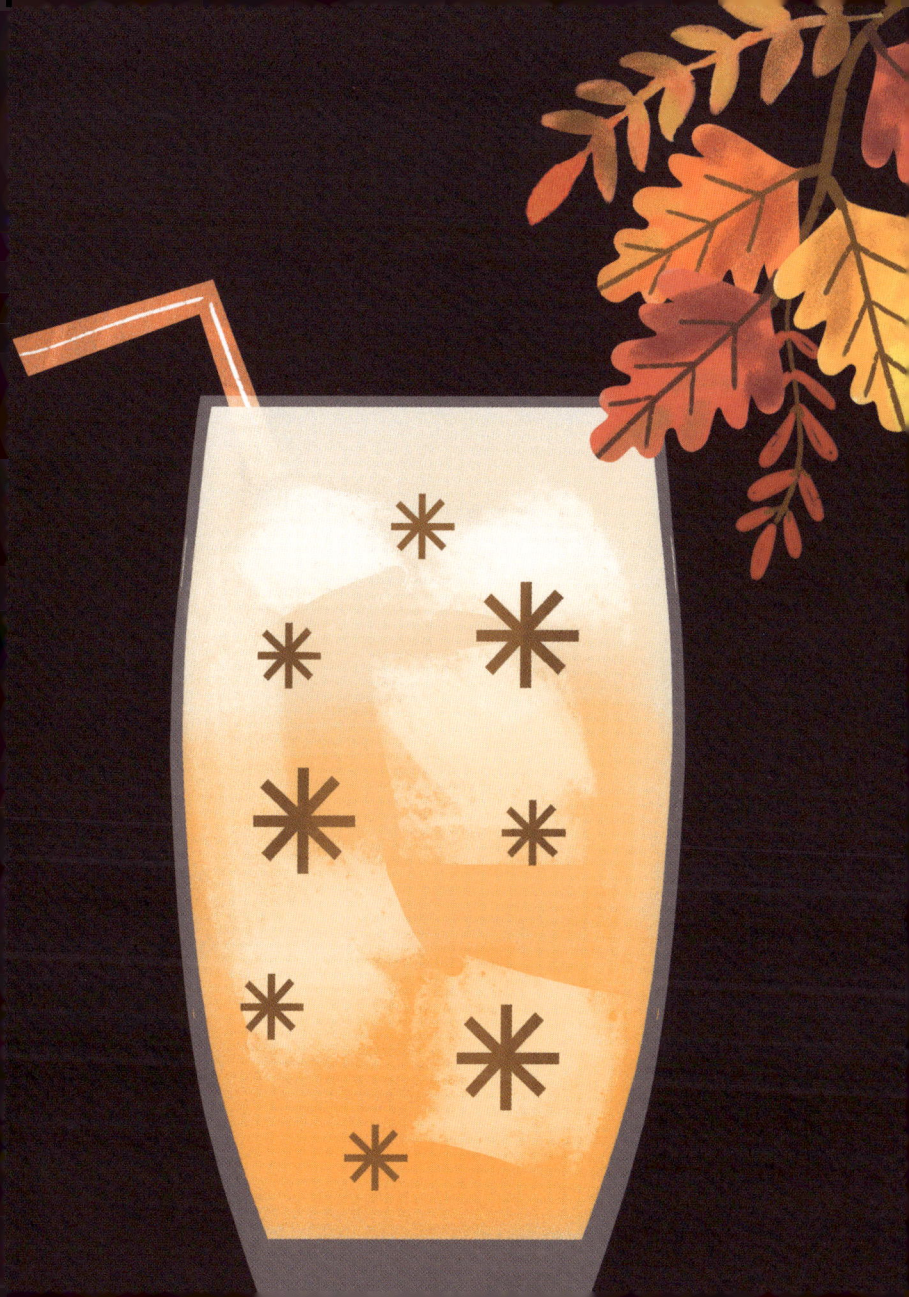

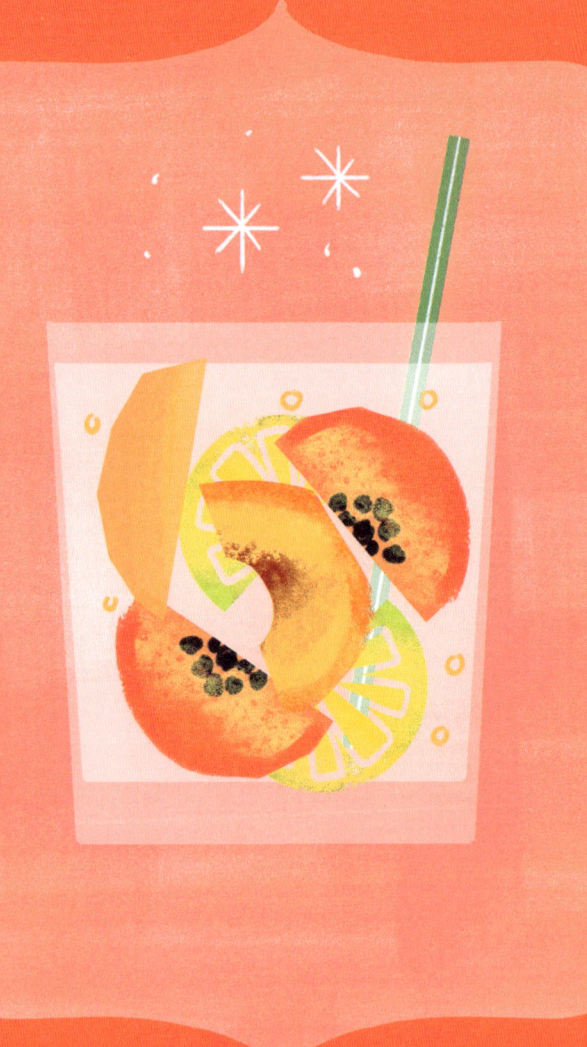

DIY GLOW WATER

There's a certain premise behind Glow Water that it is designed to enhance the drinker's skin, and hold all sorts of beneficial properties, including electrolytes that the body needs. Oh, and it's supposed to glow under a black light! When creating this drink at home, you'll simply add a bunch of fresh fruits to a glass and top it with tonic water. In this recipe, I chose the electrolyte-rich combination of mango, papaya, apricot and lemon – but you can play around with any fresh fruit combination you like. Strawberries and melons are fabulous for summer, and muddled pomegranate with an apple slice or two can turn this into a cold-weather drink. Why does this beverage glow? The quinine (responsible for tonic water's dry taste) creates a brilliant blue colour when viewed under a black light. Other soft drinks (particularly lemon-lime) have a similar, though less defined, effect. You really don't need a special light to enjoy Glow Water – the refreshing aspects of this fruit-infused water are perfect at any time of day, under any light conditions.

Serves 1

2 slices fresh mango, papaya, apricot and lemon (see headnote)
1 tbsp honey or agave nectar
ice cubes
120–180ml ounces tonic water

Add the fruits and honey (or nectar) to a large tumbler, and muddle well (to speed up the infusion process). Fill with the ice cubes, top with tonic water, then stir with vigour.

VARIATIONS

Switch to lemon-lime soda, if you like, but cut the sweetener in half, as most of those drinks are sweeter than tonic. Alternatively, use ginger-infused Simple Syrup (see page 86) instead of honey or nectar. When it comes to the fresh fruits, use any that are in season!

ORANGE FIZZ

Think of the Orange Fizz as a Mimosa meets ice cream float!
It is as delicious as it sounds, looks stunning in the glass and is an
incredibly easy mocktail to mix up. Orange sorbet is the base of
this recipe – bonus points may be earned if you manage to make it
yourself! The fizz comes from a non-alcoholic sparkling wine, and I
do encourage you to seek out a drier option because the ice cream
is already so sweet. In particular, look for non-alcoholic sparkling
wines that say 'brut' on the label. If you don't see that word, carefully
read the wine's description for any indication of a drier profile. Sweet
wines will be just a little too much on top of the sorbet. If the wine
options fail, you can always go with a sparkling water topper instead;
citrus-flavoured sparkling waters work really nicely in this drink.

Serves 1

1–2 scoops orange
  sorbet (see headnote)
120ml non-alcoholic,
  dry sparkling wine
  or citrus-flavoured
  sparkling water
1 orange slice, to garnish

Add 1 or 2 scoops of orange sorbet to
a champagne flute. Top with the wine
and garnish with the orange slice.

VARIATIONS

Replace the orange sorbet with lime
sorbet, then bring back the orange
flavour by splitting the wine with an
equal amount of freshly-squeezed
orange juice.

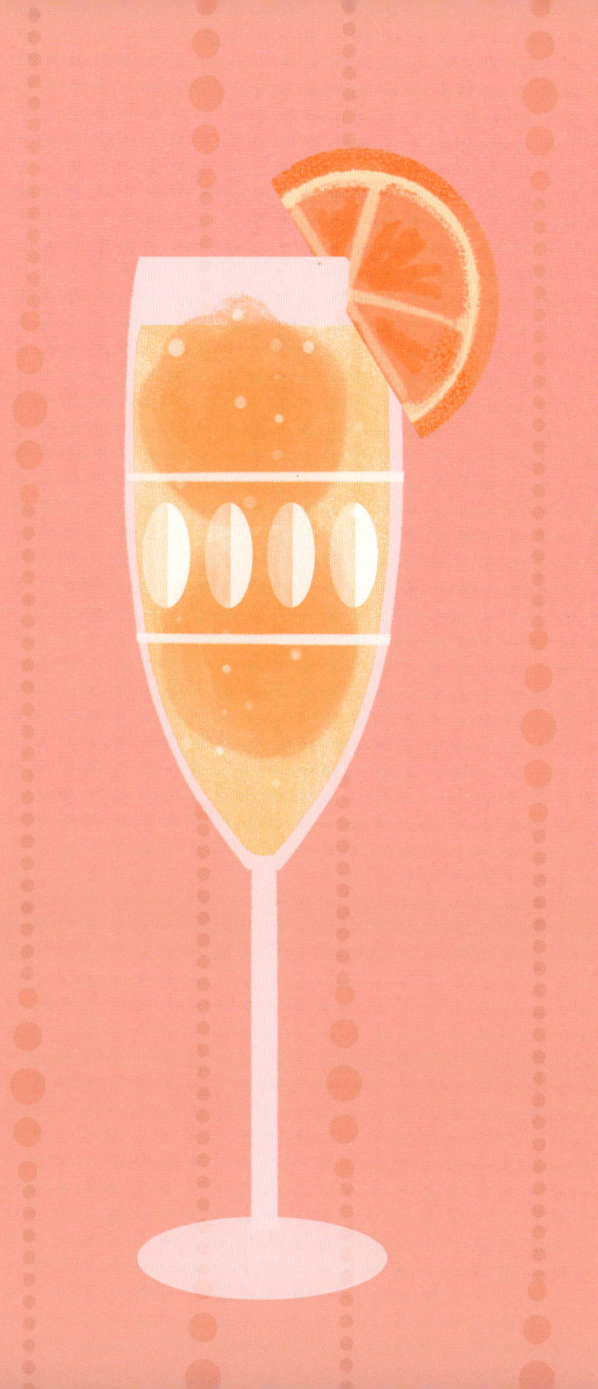

CAN'T BEET BRUNCH MOCKTAIL

While nutritious and delicious on its own, beetroot juice is a surprisingly delightful drinks mixer. When you really want to impress brunch guests (or just enjoy a tasty beverage with your eggs Benedict, on your own), this recipe is sure to please. For the Can't Beet Brunch Mocktail, I really like a zero-proof whisky. Other non-alcoholic spirits make good alternatives, though they tend to be too light to hold up against the heavy taste of the beetroot juice. Fresh lemon juice is required, while Honey Syrup provides the finishing touch to this well-balanced drink.

Serves 1

1 tbsp fresh dill
20ml Honey Syrup
  (see page 14)
15ml freshly-squeezed
  lemon juice
ice cubes
60ml zero-proof whisky
30ml beetroot juice
1 dill sprig and 1 lemon
  twist, to garnish

Muddle the dill, Honey Syrup and lemon juice in a cocktail shaker. Fill it with the ice, add the whisky and beetroot juice. Shake vigorously. Strain into a chilled cocktail glass or an old-fashioned glass over fresh ice cubes and garnish with a dill sprig and lemon twist.

VARIATIONS

Replace the Honey Syrup with maple syrup or agave nectar, cutting the pour by about half. In terms of the herbs, thyme and tarragon are pretty good substitutes for dill in this drink.

CRANBERRY–MAPLE–ROSEMARY SIPPER

On a chilly night, you'll likely want a drink that is comforting, smooth and perfectly warming. It's evenings like that when you'll be happy to have a mug full of this Cranberry-maple-rosemary Sipper. First, you'll create a cinnamon-and-rosemary-infused syrup to combine with the cranberry juice. Similar to Honey Syrup, watering down maple syrup makes it a little easier to mix into drinks, and it softens the sweetness of it. While you can simply shake maple syrup and water in a jar until the syrup dissolves, this one requires a bit of applied heat because it's also infused with the fresh rosemary. With the syrup prepared, you'll build the drink. If you haven't yet enjoyed a warm soft drink, you might be very surprised by how much you like it. I recommend trying it with one of the darker fizzy drinks: cola, root beer – or something like Dr Pepper. Heat it gently on the hob and enjoy the magic as you pour it over the sweetened cranberry juice.

Serves 1

60ml fizzy drink (see
  headnote for options)
30ml Cinnamon-
  rosemary-maple
  Syrup (see page 16)
60ml cranberry juice
1 rosemary sprig and
  1 cinnamon stick,
  to garnish

In a small saucepan, heat the fizzy drink over a low heat – just until warm. Pour the syrup and cranberry juice into a mug or Irish coffee glass, then top with the warm drink. Garnish with the rosemary sprig and cinnamon stick.

VARIATIONS

Serve this drink cold: pour the ingredients over ice, switching to a lighter fizzy drink (soda water, lemon-lime or sparkling water), if you fancy.

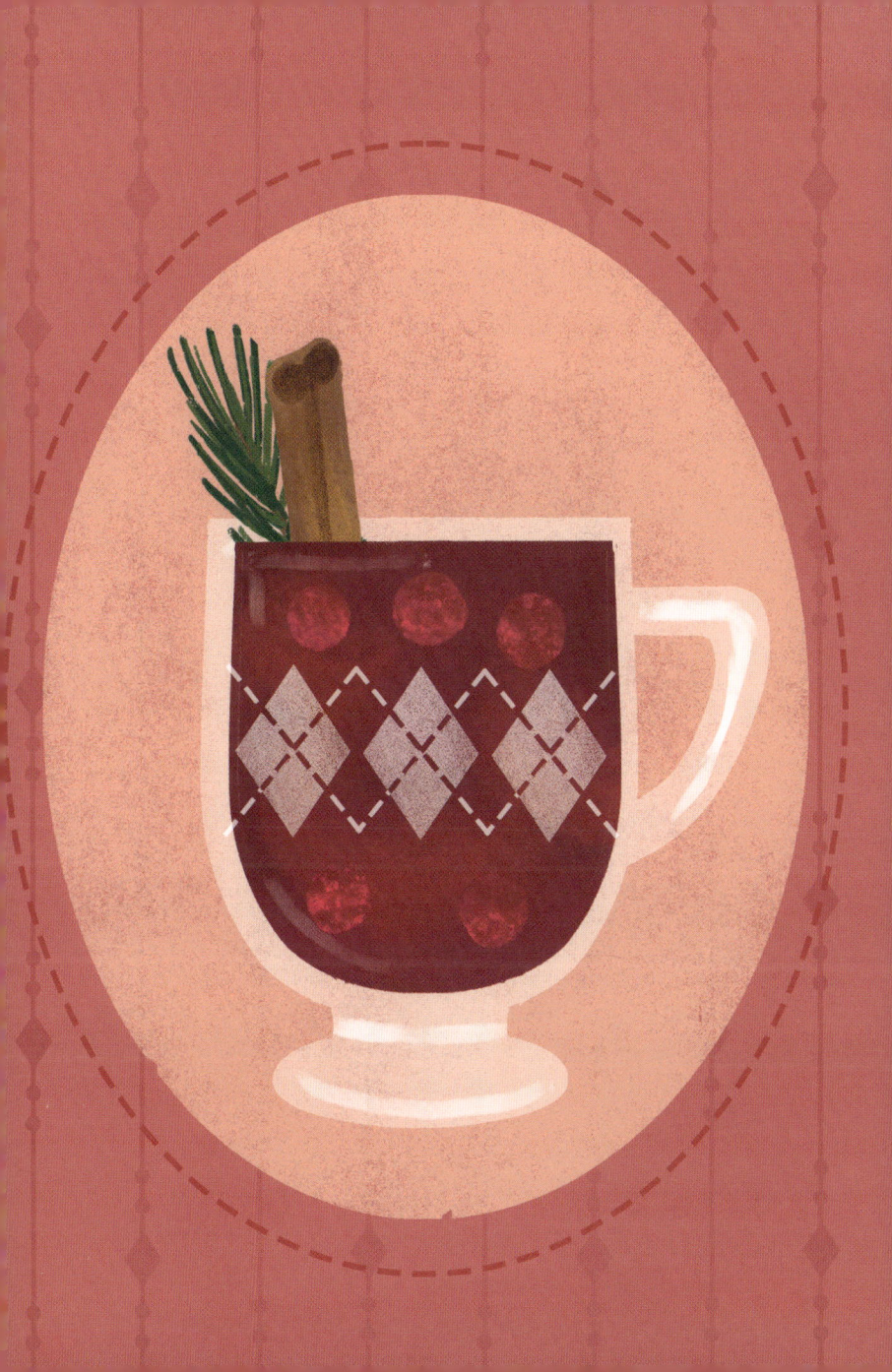

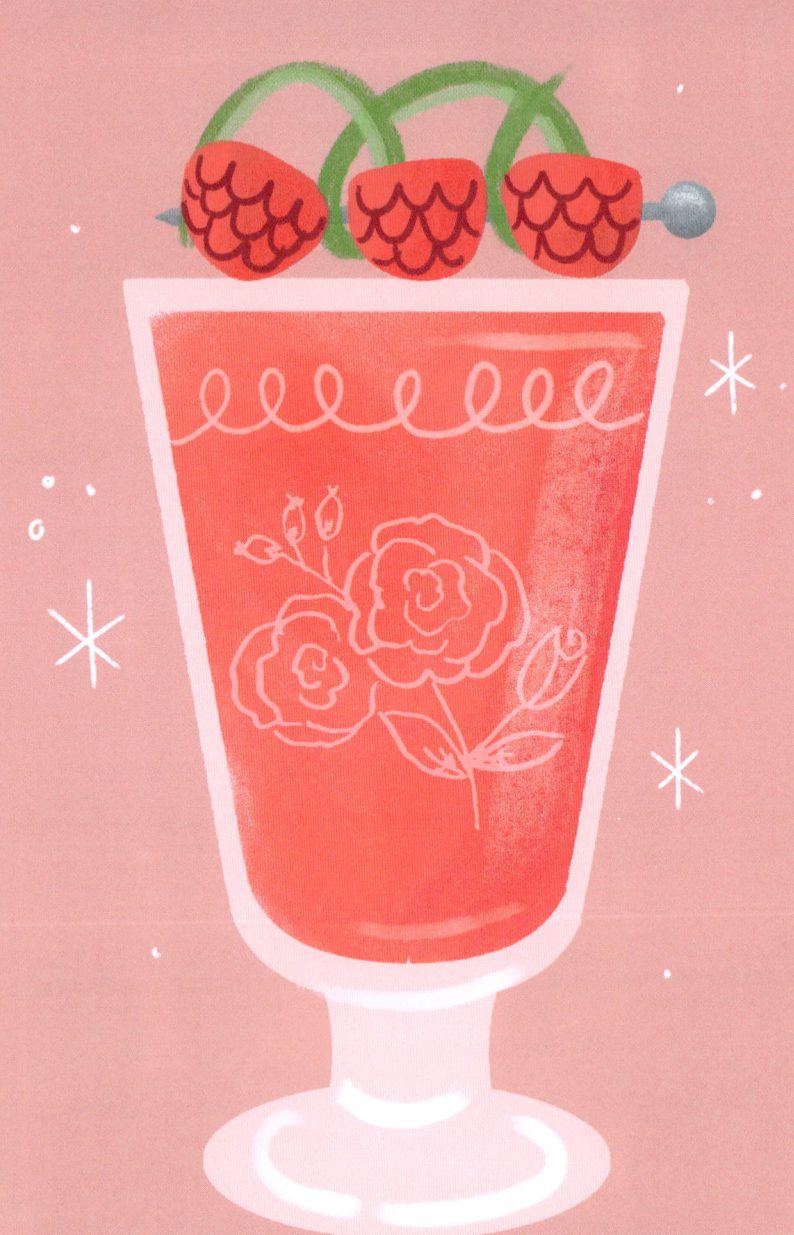

RASPBERRY AND ROSE REFRESHER

Sweet raspberries are a perfect match for the lovely floral flavour of the rose. Backed by a non-alcoholic botanical spirit, the duo come together to create a delicate and inviting mocktail. Go with a soft floral or citrus non-alcoholic spirit on this one, so that it doesn't overpower the rose. Making the Rose Syrup is as easy as any other, preferably using brown sugar rather than white – as it gives the mixer a deeper background.

Serves 1

6 fresh raspberries
30ml freshly-squeezed
  lime juice
30ml Rose Syrup
  (see page 15)
60ml zero-proof gin
  or non-alcoholic
  botanical spirit
ice cubes
1 lime twist and 3 fresh
  raspberries, to garnish

Into a cocktail shaker, add the 6 raspberries, lime juice and Rose Syrup. Muddle well to crush the berries. Add the spirit and fill with the ice. Shake well, then strain into a chilled cocktail glass and garnish with the lime twist and a few fresh raspberries.

G 'N' TEA SOUR

It's always fun to play around in the bar and give a familiar drink a new spin – the results here are rather interesting. As with any sour cocktail, citrus and syrup are a must. To give this drink a floral touch, I've opted for either Rose Syrup or Lavender-honey Syrup. You'll also want to brew your best green tea a little stronger than you normally would (add extra leaves or steep it for a few additional minutes). For the non-alcoholic botanical spirit, I like the lighter options, although some of the juniper-forward non-alcoholic gins are rather interesting. And, finally, kombucha! This fizzy, acidic drink is an intriguing alternative to other fizzy drinks, and you can choose a fruity kombucha if you like.

Serves 1

ice cubes
30ml freshly-squeezed
  lemon juice
30ml Rose Syrup
  (see page 15) or
  Lavender-honey Syrup
  (see page 14)
60ml chilled green tea
60ml zero-proof gin
  or non-alcoholic
  botanical spirit
30ml kombucha
1 lemon slice and
  3 maraschino cherries,
  to garnish

Into a cocktail shaker filled with the ice, pour the lemon juice, syrup, tea and spirit. Shake well, strain into an old-fashioned glass over fresh ice cubes, then top with the kombucha. Garnish with the lemon slice and maraschino cherries.

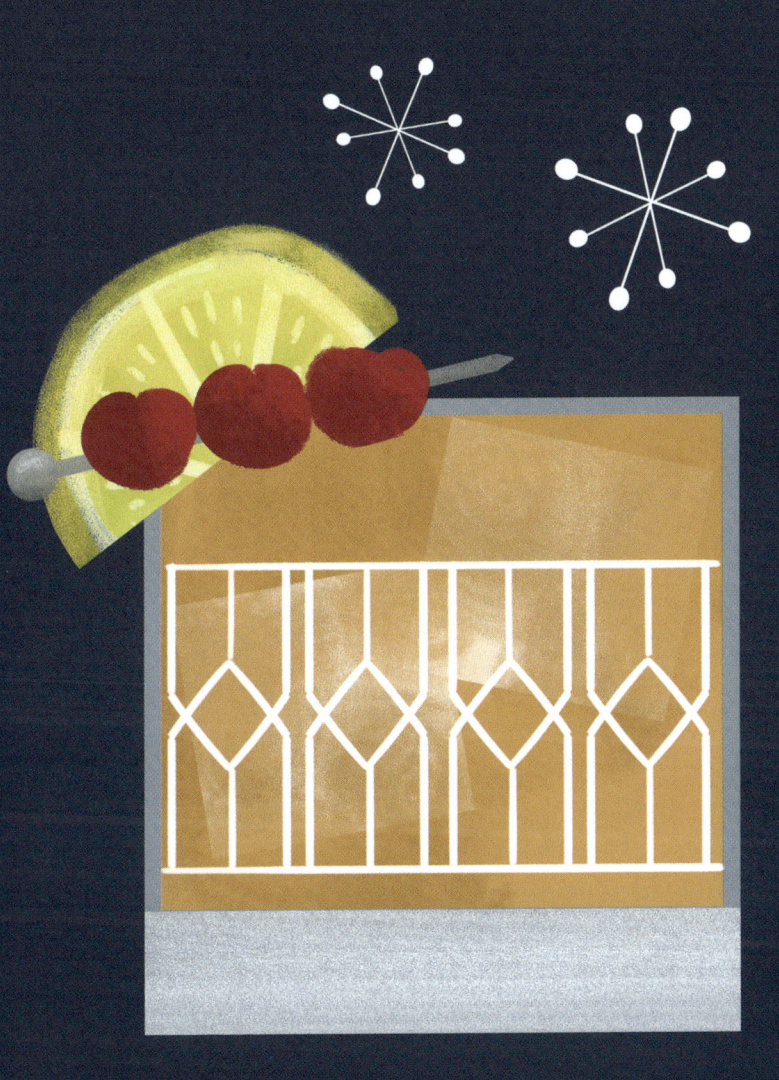

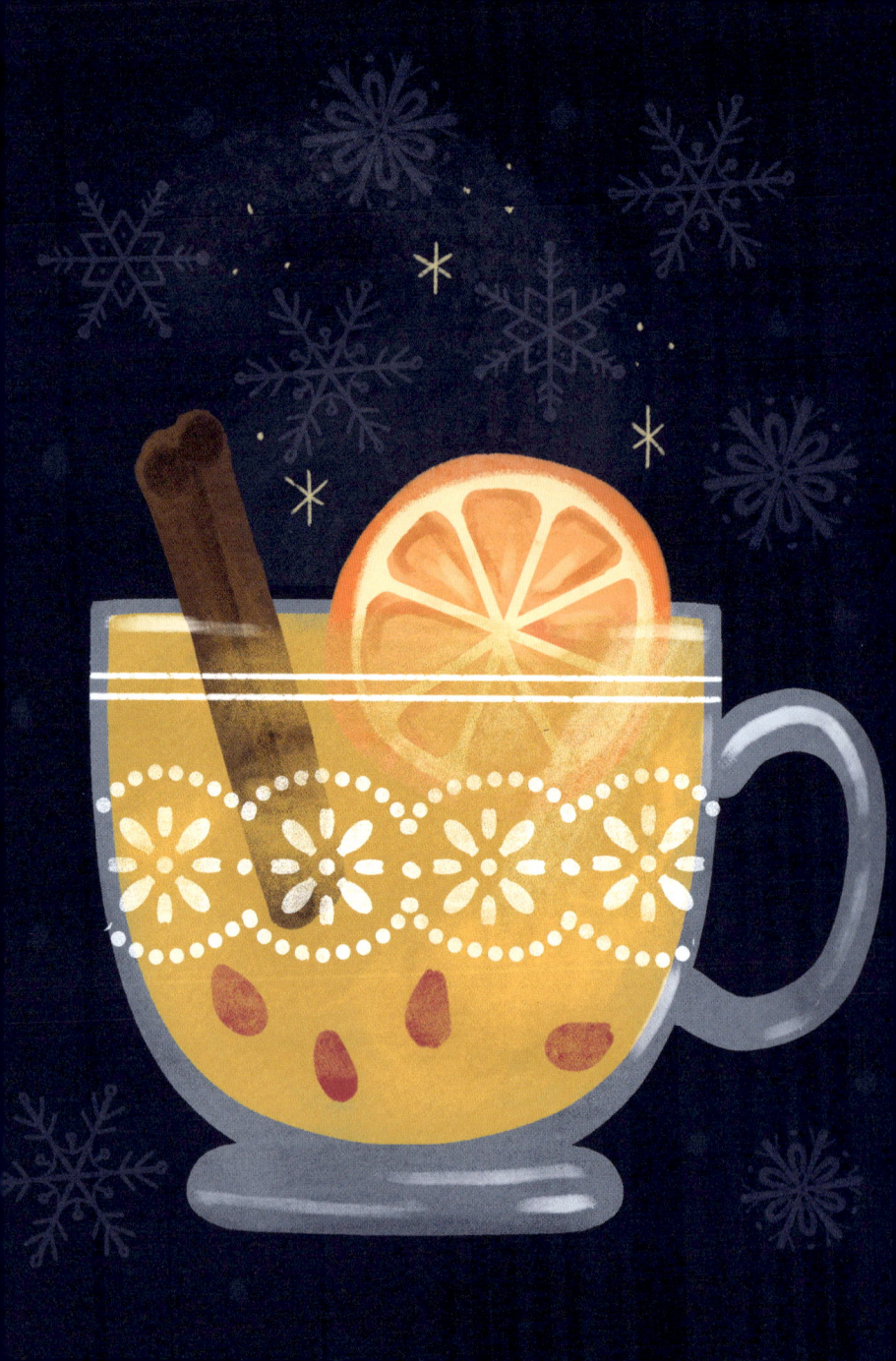

WARMING WINTER CUP

As refreshing as the Summer Cup Mocktail (see page 97), this Winter Cup is designed to be an aromatic warm drink that celebrates the best fruits of the cooler season. Rather than cucumber and strawberries, this one relies on pomegranate and spiced syrup. You might even think of this one as a toddy. It is a lovely drink. Orange remains in this cup, though it's accented with fresh pomegranate arils, and brewed green tea adds a lovely accent. To bring it all together, you'll make a brown sugar Simple Syrup that includes all those favourite, warming spices of the season. Add a shot of zero-proof whisky, rum – or even gin – if you prefer, as any of them will only add to the drink's complexity.

Serves 1

2 orange slices
40g pomegranate arils
15ml spiced brown sugar
  syrup (see Simple Syrup
  variations, pages 12–13)
60ml apple cider
60ml brewed hot
  green tea
45ml zero-proof whisky,
  rum or gin (optional)
1 orange slice and
  1 cinnamon stick,
  to garnish

In a ceramic mug or heatproof glass mug, muddle the orange, pomegranate and syrup to release the fruits' juices. Top with the cider and hot green tea, add your zero-proof spirit of choice, then garnish the drink with the orange slice and cinnamon stick.

INDEX

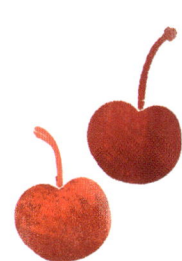

CREDITS

About the author

Colleen Graham is a seasoned mixologist who has researched and written about cocktails and mixed drinks for well over a decade. Sharing her passion for crafting a great beverage, she brings her Midwest practicality into the mix to prove that, by borrowing a few tips and tricks that bartenders have used for over a century, anyone can create a drink that is sure to impress. She is also an avid gardener and the author of *Rosé Made Me Do It* and *Vodka Made Me Do It*.

Acknowledgements

From Colleen: I must thank my husband, Shannon, for his support and willingness to be an honest taste tester during countless drink experiments. I hope the book's recipes inspire you to create your own concoctions. This is just the beginning of the no- and lo-alcohol revolution. Explore new 'spirits' and mixers, grab fresh produce – or grow your own – and start mixing. The possibilities are endless. The journey is exciting! Even a 'bad' drink can lead to something spectacular.

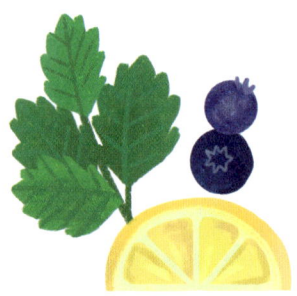